Managing AIDS
in the Workplace

Managing AIDS in the Workplace

Sam B. Puckett, LL.B., M.B.A. and
Alan R. Emery, Ph.D.

Addison-Wesley Publishing Company, Inc.
Reading, Massachusetts   Menlo Park, California
New York   Don Mills, Ontario
Wokingham, England   Amsterdam   Bonn
Sydney   Singapore   Tokyo   Madrid
San Juan

Library of Congress Cataloging-in-Publication Data

Puckett, Sam B.
  Managing AIDS in the workplace / by Sam B. Puckett and Alan R. Emery
  p.   cm.
  Includes index.
  ISBN 0-201-08058-3
    1. AIDS (Disease)—Social aspects.   2. AIDS (Disease)—Law and
  legislation.   3. Employee rights.   4. Industrial hygiene.
  I. Emery, Alan R.   II. Title.
  RC607.A26P835   1988
  658.3'8—dc 19   88-10492
                                                                          CIP

Jacket design by Robert Lowe
Text design by Joyce C. Weston
Set in 11-point Bembo by Neil W. Kelley

ABCDEFGHIJ-DO-898

First printing, May 1988

CONTENTS

PREFACE

Since 1984, we have had the privilege of working with many of the nation's leading corporations, as well as with both small and large organizations of all types, in their efforts to develop cost-effective, legal and humane approaches to the complicated challenge of AIDS in the workplace. Our purpose in writing this book is to share with you what managers in organizations of all types, sizes and locations have learned about managing the AIDS epidemic. Our goal is to assist you in "managing" AIDS in the workplace in a way that protects your organization, conforms with the law, treats all employees fairly and equally and contributes towards the saving of lives and the ending of the AIDS epidemic.

Despite the many fears still associated with this disease, managers planning for the issue of AIDS in the workplace, or actually facing this issue at the moment, have several significant advantages over those who had to face it as far back as 1981:

- The public health Guidelines regarding AIDS in the workplace are clear, consistent and widely accepted among both the scientific and business communities. Despite continuing public fears about the disease, the mysteries of AIDS are largely resolved. There is considerable scientific agreement about the means by which AIDS is and is not transmitted. There is a solid basis for confidence that people with AIDS do not pose a threat in the workplace, either to co-workers or to customers.

- AIDS is no longer considered to be a new disease. Since 1984, federal regulations have required that every case of AIDS diagnosed anywhere in America be reported to the Centers for Disease Control. Tens of thousands of cases have been analyzed in this country, and thousands studied in Canada, England, Europe, Australia, New Zealand and other countries. There is widespread cooperation among epidemiologists—the scientists responsible for the study of epidemics—in most major countries of the world. In face, AIDS is one of the most widely studied diseases in history.

▪ A multitude of models now exist for managing AIDS in a variety of workplace settings. While AIDS in the workplace may seem to many to be a relatively new issue, many organizations have been encountering cases of AIDS in one fashion or another ever since the first ones were identified in 1981. Various approaches have been tried. At this point in the course of the epidemic, companies of every size in all industries in all parts of the country have made decisions about AIDS. Some good decisions have led to constructive results, and some bad decisions have brought on embarrassing legal and financial disasters.

▪ Although there remain some open questions regarding the legal obligations of employers to workers diagnosed with AIDS, the general direction of the law is now clear. There is considerable agreement among labor lawyers about the status of AIDS within the meaning of handicap legislation. Several cities and some states now have laws specifically applicable to AIDS. Some prohibit discrimination against people with AIDS; others deal specifically with pre-employment screening for AIDS, or with the confidentiality of antibody test results.

▪ Although irrational employee reactions to AIDS are still possible, the experience of most organizations is that, when life and death issues are involved, human compassion, when given an opportunity to come forth, inevitably triumphs over irrational fear. Underneath it all, most employees are basically reasonable, caring and concerned about the well-being of others. When those concerns are nurtured, and when the relevant facts are presented clearly and calmly, employees will generally cooperate in situations involving AIDS, even though there is likely to remain a sense of apprehension at some level about the disease. Also, most workers appreciate it when employers provide honest information about subjects like this.

- Despite its deadly and incurable nature, AIDS is a preventable disease. Moreover, most Americans can avoid completely any exposure to AIDS, now that the methods of transmission and prevention are well known. You and your employees—and your family and children—can do so as well. The potential cost to your company health plan could be horrendous; but it can be controlled through provision of a plan for preventive education for insured workers and their covered dependents and by case management of medical costs. Education and prevention are the most cost-effective responses to this epidemic.

- AIDS, despite its medical and scientific focus, involves issues with which management is already familiar and experienced. You will find that you know how to deal with most aspects of AIDS in the workplace. Once you have the facts and an accurate perspective on the disease, and you understand the real issues underlying employee reactions to AIDS, you simply need to act, based on what you already know.

Socio-political aspects of AIDS make it difficult for the government and the public health sector to deal with the epidemic. Moreover, there are psychological factors responsible for management's reluctance to manage AIDS in the workplace. To a certain extent, of course, procrastination is a common human tendency, and setting priorities requires putting aside the non-immediate problem. Planning for a future issue requires finding time to do so in the midst of today's crises. It is easy to find reasons to avoid planning for AIDS in your organization, and we're confident that you are capable of finding even better excuses than the ones we've heard before.

This book will give you a chance to consider why management often resists dealing with the issue of AIDS until the organization faces a crisis over an actual or perceived case of the disease. In our experience, all of the perceived pitfalls and fears surrounding AIDS in the workplace, and all the justifications for procrastinating about it, can be avoided through careful planning.

If you are the person being asked to "manage" AIDS in your workplace, or if you recognize your own responsibility to promote a planned response to AIDS within your organization, it is important that you have a clear understanding of what this disease is, what causes it, how it works in the human body, how it is transmitted from person to person and how it is *not* transmitted. It is also useful to understand the prognosis for this disease in the future. Please be assured that managers are capable of understanding this disease and deciding how to prepare for it. Medical training and a scientific background are not necessary to understand AIDS, to intelligently explain it to others or to decide how your organization will deal with the epidemic.

We hope that our book will help you to recognize the need to plan for AIDS as a potential issue for your organization, to examine the experiences of others, to consider your options in the context of your own corporate culture and to determine the most appropriate course of action for your company. In addition, we hope you come to understand that:

- Employees with AIDS do not pose a threat to other employees or to customers in the workplace.

- AIDS *cannot* be transmitted during normal social or occupational interactions. Thus, there is no logical basis for treating AIDS on the job any differently from the way you would treat other life-threatening illness such as cancer, stroke or heart disease.

- Education resolves irrational fears about AIDS. Ultimately, workers respond well to educational programs about AIDS. In fact, employees appreciate management's facing controversial issues in an honest, straightforward manner.

- AIDS is manageable. Preparation and planning avoid potential pitfalls and make possible an AIDS response that complies with the law, maintains rationality in the workplace, treats all employees with dignity and respect and minimizes the cost to the organization of this new epidemic.

Sam Puckett
Alan Emery
San Francisco
March, 1988

INTRODUCTION

by Robert D. Haas, President and Chief Executive Officer
Levi Strauss & Co.

Events take on special meaning when they touch us personally.

I remember quite clearly when AIDS, as a health issue, a human issue, and a business issue, took on that kind of meaning for me.

The year was 1982. Several employees asked for permission to distribute literature about AIDS in the lobby of our headquarters building in San Francisco. I was stunned by the reaction they got from many of their co-workers. Some were frightened they might contract the disease just by talking to someone who was concerned about the issue. Others assumed that the employees distributing literature must be gay, because AIDS had been identified as primarily a disease striking gay and bisexual men.

I didn't know a good deal about AIDS at that time. But I understood two things right away. First, this was an issue that would touch all of us, and second, as a company executive, it was my responsibility to help set standards about how we would respond.

I asked to join the group and invited other senior managers to work with us. For several days, we took turns staffing an information booth in our lobby at lunchtime, handing out information about AIDS and how it is—and is not—transmitted.

That was six years ago. Since then, AIDS has become an epidemic and taken a terrible toll. We have lost many friends. As employers we have also had to confront serious business consequences as well—the loss of talented employees, the enormous medical and insurance costs, the disruption in the workforce, the fear, prejudice, and discrimination that often occur.

Although these issues are complex, they are still manageable. I believe it is our responsibility as business leaders to manage as carefully and as compassionately as we can. For no matter what business we're in, all of us depend on the talents, productivity, and goodwill of our employees. They are an asset we can safeguard through open, honest communications.

Through our efforts at Levi Strauss & Co., and our experiences with other companies, I've come to the conclusion that there are three keys to successful management of AIDS in the workplace.

First, companies must address AIDS in a compassionate, responsible, and humane manner. AIDS, or any other life-threatening disease, can rob its victims of life, work, and human contact. As employers, we are responsible for making sure employees are treated with respect and dignity.

The law will eventually compel employers to face the issues surrounding AIDS. I think, as senior managers, we should not wait to be compelled. AIDS is not somebody else's problem. It is a community problem, and community business leaders have an important part to play in solving it.

Second, at Levi Strauss & Co., we've seen that education is the key to building, understanding, and changing attitudes. By educating yourself and your employees about AIDS, you can reduce the impact the disease will have in the workplace. Education can minimize, if not eliminate, prejudice and unwarranted fear about AIDS.

Today, fewer than one in ten American companies have an AIDS program or policy. That brings me to the third key approach to managing this issue. The impetus must come from the top. In any organization it is the senior managers who must support and encourage the development of sound AIDS policies and programs.

We must pay more than lip service to these programs—we must make them corporate as well as personal priorities. We have to be visible in our support of human resource professionals as they attempt to deal with AIDS-related problems. We need to recognize the critical role Employee Assistance Programs can play, and we should talk about these issues with business leaders from other companies.

AIDS is a moving target. The research and clinical communities are scrambling to learn more, try new ideas, and explore new treatments. We must make sure that in any business relationships we have with the health and human services community, we guarantee access to that knowledge.

There are many tests of a company's character—quality of goods and services, position in the marketplace, public reputation. I feel that the issue of AIDS in the workplace is one such test. Employees will watch; the public will watch. They want to know if American business is capable of responding effectively and compassionately.

To that end, think of this book as much more than information. It should be a manual, a working document to help you and your colleagues manage the business aspects of this medical and social tragedy.

I believe we are equal to the task. We cannot afford, in either business terms or human terms, to fail.

1 ‖ The AIDS Epidemic and the Workplace

For more than a decade, a new and deadly virus has been spreading across the United States, Canada, England, western Europe, Australia and virtually every other country of the world. It was not until 1981 that there was any hint of its passage, and it was 1984 before the virus was even identified. Its precise origins remain obscure; its ultimate impact on society is necessarily still a matter of conjecture. By the 1990s, however, this new virus will have killed tens of thousands of people and infected millions of others, creating an international public health crisis of historic magnitude. AIDS has become the object of political controversy, and an expensive and awkward issue for organizations of all kinds.

The AIDS virus made its first appearance during the 1960s or perhaps earlier in several countries of south central Africa. The virus is one of a particular class of viruses—known as "retroviruses"—of which only a handful have ever been discovered, and which prior to the 1980s were thought to cause such diseases as cancer and leukemia in animals. This new form of retrovirus has been named by its various discoverers as "Human T-Lymphotropic Virus Type III" ("HTLV-3"), "Lymphadenopathy Associated Virus" ("LAV") and "AIDS Retro Virus" ("ARV"). In 1986 an international scientific committee gave it the official designation

1

"Human Immunodeficiency Virus," or "HIV." To the public it is known as "the AIDS virus," and the medical condition it causes is known as "AIDS"—*Acquired Immune Deficiency Syndrome.*

In the early months of 1981, physicians in Los Angeles, New York and San Francisco unknowingly encountered the first manifestations of a new and deadly medical phenomenon. Young male patients in their twenties and thirties, obviously seriously ill, were presenting with diseases seldom encountered by the general practitioner. Some of these patients had pneumocystis pneumonia, an unusual lung disease caused by a protozoan, which results in the patient suffocating as the lungs become filled with fluid. Other patients had Kaposi's sarcoma, an extremely rare cancer of the capillaries and a condition previously found only in old men of Mediterranean descent. These patients had other diseases not normally seen in combination and had experienced profound weight loss and general debilitation. Some were near death.

The physicians were perplexed, as were the specialists to whom they referred their patients for treatment. At the time, none of these doctors could know that these few patients represented the beginning of a medical challenge that would change their practice, change their lives and alter the course of medical history, if not history in general. Uncertain as to either the underlying cause or the recommended course of treatment of the patients' conditions, some of the doctors contacted the Centers for Disease Control (CDC) in Atlanta, the huge unit of the United States Public Health Service responsible for tracking the course and incidence of diseases, to ask if they had encountered anything like this before.

Upon receiving independent reports of similar medical anomalies from three cities within a short period of time, officials at the CDC speculated that something new and potentially significant was afoot. To alert physicians and health departments, a short bulletin about the physicians' reports was published in the CDC's "Weekly Morbidity and Mortality Report," the official medical scorecard of the nation's health. A terse one-paragraph report from the CDC to the medical community in mid-1981 was the first of what would become a flood of such reports over the succeeding months.

This book is not only about the presence and impact of AIDS in the workplace but it is also about opportunities for saving lives. We have written the book for managers who are concerned about managing the consequences of this epidemic in the workplace. Overseeing the consequences of an epidemic is not normally thought of as a management function. It is unlikely that this topic could have been found in the curricula of the nation's graduate schools of business administration even a short time ago. It is unlikely that the men and women who manage the tens of thousands of organizations in our society—business organizations, nonprofit organizations, government agencies—received any formal academic training in the management of epidemics.

Nevertheless, to a large degree, management is the art of dealing effectively with the environment in which the organization finds itself. Many organizations over the past decade have found themselves suddenly coping with the spectre of AIDS within their environment; many more organizations will be in the position of having to face some aspect of AIDS during the next decade. Overseeing this particular aspect of the organizational environment may well become part of *your* responsibility at some point within the next several years. How well you manage that aspect of your organizational environment will considerably influence your organization's medical and legal costs, its public and employee relations, its efficiency and stability. It will also influence your own career.

By mid-1988, seven years after the first cases of AIDS were reported to public health officials, more than 60,000 Americans had already been diagnosed with the disease. More than half of those diagnosed had died; for the others, death seems only a matter of time. The life expectancy after a diagnosis of AIDS averages only eighteen months. There is no cure for the condition and no

The Chronology of AIDS	
1960–70s (?)	AIDS virus originates (?) in Africa.
1977	AIDS virus arrives in New York.
1978	AIDS virus arrives in Los Angeles and San Francisco.
1981	First medical cases reported to CDC.
1982	First organization on AIDS created in New York.
1983	The name "AIDS" established.
1984	The "AIDS virus" discovered: Pasteur (France) announces LAV; Gallo (USA) announces HTLV–3; Levy (USA) announces ARV.
1985	U.S. government declares AIDS "top health priority"; predicts AIDS vaccine ready within six months.
1985	CDC issues Guidelines for AIDS in the Workplace.
1986	Surgeon General issues report on AIDS.
1987	Virus renamed "HIV" (Human Immuno-deficiency Virus).
1987	Presidential Commission on AIDS appointed.
1988	AIDS diagnoses in the U.S. surpass 60,000; 50 new cases added each working day; no cure or vaccine in sight.

vaccine to prevent its spread. Only the most optimistic researchers expect to achieve the necessary scientific breakthroughs required for a medical solution to AIDS before the end of the century.

During 1988, AIDS cases were being diagnosed in the U.S. at the rate of more than 50 new cases each working day. There were cases of AIDS in all major American cities and in all fifty states. Every day during 1988, more than 25 Americans died of AIDS. During the same time, the demographics of those being diagnosed with AIDS were beginning to change.

Nearly three-fourths of cumulative AIDS cases are still found among homosexual or bisexual men, with about one-fifth of cases diagnosed among intravenous (IV) drug-users—mostly because of the overwhelmingly high rates of initial infection within those populations from the earliest days of the epidemic. But the percentage of cases diagnosed among heterosexuals, women, infants, teenagers and minorities was increasing proportionately faster. The most recent statistical projections predict slow but long-term changes in the AIDS patient population. Of particular concern during the same time frame was the recognition that ethnic minorities, particularly Blacks and Hispanics, were contracting AIDS at a rate twice that of their numbers within the population. Cases of AIDS among newborn infants, a strikingly expanding group for the disease, were found most often among the offspring of Black and Hispanic women who became infected with the AIDS virus before or during pregnancy. Concern was also growing among both parents and health officials about the risk of AIDS among teenagers of all races and all economic levels, considering the almost inevitable tendency of adolescents to experiment with sex and drugs, the fundamental means by which AIDS is spread.

In the few cities hardest hit by the AIDS epidemic—New York, Newark, San Francisco, Los Angeles, Miami, Chicago, Houston, Washington, D.C.—health care delivery systems are increasingly taxed to provide medical care and other necessary support to people with AIDS. Every public health and medical expert projecting the future of the epidemic has reached the same conclusion—AIDS is growing rapidly, and the situation will only become far worse. The San Francisco Department of Public Health, for example, projected in mid-1987 that the cost of AIDS cases by the end of the decade would exceed the total existing budget of all services provided by San Francisco General Hospital. Health officials in New York and New Jersey have warned of potential bankruptcy for their states' public health systems from the projected burden of AIDS.

Even more frightening and of considerable concern to employers, the CDC estimated that by 1986, between one and two million Americans had already been infected with the virus that causes AIDS and are at risk for eventually developing the fatal conditions associated with long-term infection by the virus. In the meantime, those people are also capable of passing the virus on to others, thereby expanding the scope of the epidemic. In the absence of the massive education and prevention efforts that many experts have called for, only the virus's very limited means of transmission has prevented a much larger public health disaster.

While no one knows how many of the one to two million people who are infected with the AIDS virus will eventually develop the full fatal form of the disease, the U.S. Public Health Service has concluded that well over one-quarter of a million Americans will develop AIDS by the end of 1991. However, the estimate does not include the much larger number of people who would require medical care for AIDS-related Complex (ARC), an AIDS-like condition that is also caused by the AIDS virus but that does not quite meet the CDC's technical definition of AIDS.

By the beginning of 1992, American deaths from the AIDS epidemic are expected to reach roughly three times the number of deaths of all American service personnel in the Viet Nam War. According to CDC-sponsored studies, the projected medical costs of these U.S. cases alone will reach $8.5 billion in 1991. Much of the medical costs will be borne by employer-paid health plans and may transform this traditional and widely accepted part of American working life. Indirect costs attributable to premature loss of worker productivity due to AIDS-related illness or early death in the U.S. alone are estimated to rise from $7.0 billion in 1986 to $55.6 billion in 1991.*

---

*Institute for Health Policy Studies, University of California San Francisco Medical Center, "Estimates of the Direct and Indirect Costs of AIDS in the United States." *Public Health Reports*, January/February 1987.

The World Health Organization (WHO) has found cases of AIDS on every continent except Antarctica. Infection rates in some countries of Africa—where the virus is thought to have originated—vastly exceed infection rates in the United States, prompting fears in those countries that their already inadequate medical systems will soon be totally overwhelmed. WHO's casualty projections for Third World countries, where AIDS is equally distributed between males and females, run into the millions of potential cases. No nation is exempt; cases of AIDS have been reported even in the Soviet Union and China. AIDS is a dramatically growing, worldwide medical tragedy with no medical cure in sight. By the early 1990s, it is likely that the AIDS epidemic will be the most deadly and costly epidemic of the twentieth century. AIDS deaths will exceed the cost in lives of the forty-year-long polio epidemic, and could approach the scale of the great influenza epidemic of 1918–1919, which took 400,000 lives in the U.S. and caused millions of deaths worldwide.

As "a disease of consenting adults," AIDS is more difficult to transmit from person to person than the diseases that caused the mass epidemics of the past—influenza, typhoid, cholera, yellow fever and tuberculosis. These diseases caused epidemics that spread by "casual contact," such as sneezing or coughing. Because of the specifically limited ways in which the AIDS virus can be passed from person to person, AIDS can never become the twentieth century equivalent of the infamous bubonic plague. Nevertheless, it has become the major epidemic of our time and will probably prove to be the major worldwide epidemic of our century.

In America and throughout the world, AIDS has generated heated social and political controversy for the public health establishment as conservatives and liberals battle out longstanding differences in basic philosophy about people and government. Because cases of AIDS first appeared among homosexual men, then among users of illegal intravenous drugs, the disease became associated in the public mind with only those groups. Even as AIDS began to strike other segments of the population and to appear all over the country, it was difficult to change the public's perception that AIDS affects only "those kinds of people" who live in "those cities."

The deaths from AIDS of Rock Hudson, Liberace, Broadway producer Michael Bennett, Connecticut Republican Congressman Stewart McKinney, lawyer Roy Cohn, Washington Redskins football player Jerry Smith and others helped to give a human face to the target groups for AIDS, but the original stigma associated with sex, drugs and homosexuality remained. These public attitudes towards AIDS and the people who were identified with AIDS were sufficiently troublesome to the Surgeon General of the United States, Dr. C. Everett Koop, that, in his report to the public on AIDS he felt compelled to admonish Americans to "put those feelings behind us," and to remind them that "we are fighting a disease, not people."

It is now clear that heterosexuals who have had multiple sexual partners are at risk for AIDS, although the risk remains statistically low. Nevertheless, journalists have made "heterosexuals and AIDS" a frequent front-page story in the nation's newsmagazines. From Milwaukee to Memphis, from Boston to Bakersfield, AIDS became a topic of conversation among heterosexual singles. "Safe sex" and condoms became topics for satirical comment by cartoonists and comedians. From their television pulpits, a handful of fundamentalist evangelists championed the notion that AIDS was, after all, God's punishment on sinners of various types, and that the solution to the AIDS epidemic was simply to lock up all those who could—or who might be able to—spread the disease. Some conservative politicians were inclined to agree. Most other legislators saw AIDS as a very tricky, no-win political issue and opted to quietly distance themselves from the subject as much as possible.

What ordinarily would be a difficult medical and public health issue under the best of circumstances had become a complex con-

troversy over morals, religion and basic political philosophy regarding the rights of individuals, the role of government and the
most effective way of promoting human behavior change. As a
consequence, remarkably little action has been taken to stop a
preventable disease. AIDS funding became a game in which the
federal health agencies requested large amounts of money for AIDS
treatment and research. The requests were cut by Administration
budget officials before submission to Congress; the Congress re-
stored the cuts and even increased the amounts beyond those originally requested. The appropriations in excess of the amounts sub-
mitted by the White House were then frozen by the Office of
Management & Budget, and the money not spent. The cycle was
repeated the following year.

The Reagan administration itself became deeply divided on
strategies toward AIDS, as the 70-year-old born-again-Christian
Surgeon General, Dr. C. Everett Koop, sided with public health
officials and argued for widespread sex education and the promotion of condoms, while Secretary of Education William Bennett
marshalled support for a highly traditional stance promoting only
abstinence and marital fidelity.

In trying to promote educated behavioral change among those
who were at risk for AIDS, public health officials everywhere
found themselves once again dealing with the two health issues—
sex and drugs—about which the public health establishment had
the longest and most dismal record of failure. Barred by conservative political forces from speaking frankly and openly about sex
or drug use, and finding themselves generally distrusted by the
very audiences they were trying hardest to reach, the public health
officials of the country were caught in a difficult bind. There
seemed to be no clear path to success, and there was no political
consensus about what to do.

To further complicate matters, a generation of people unaccus-
tomed to epidemics of infectious diseases, having assumed that
medical technology has conquered epidemics forever, has reacted

with surprisingly strong and irrational fear towards the possibility of casual contagion by the AIDS virus. Despite repeated and consistent statements by public health officials that AIDS cannot be transmitted through ordinary social or workplace interactions, many people are nevertheless afraid to be in the same room with a person who has been diagnosed with AIDS, or even a person suspected of carrying the AIDS virus. As a political statement of displeasure with the groups who are associated with the disease, some people have actively promoted the fear reactions in others.

In several highly publicized events, workers confronted with the possibility of having to work alongside an AIDS patient have walked off the job. Under the glare of television lights, angry parents have picketed schools as a child with AIDS attempted to attend classes with other children. Claiming the need to protect themselves from the demonstrators, police officers patrolling AIDS political demonstrations have donned protective gloves.

Astonishingly, some members of the health care community throughout the country have reacted with greater irrationality to AIDS than has the average layperson. To knowledgeable public health officials, the frequently inappropriate response of the medical profession to AIDS is a professional embarrassment. Public statements of irrational fear made by health care providers and isolated but highly publicized instances of physicians refusing to care for AIDS patients—despite clear scientific evidence that common infection control procedures are adequate—have confused an already suspicious and frightened general public.

It is regrettable that the AIDS crisis has occurred at a time when public paranoia about government conspiracies and cover-ups has reached an all time high. Previous generations of Americans may have trusted what they were told by medical and public health officials, but the current generation is more skeptical. Mervyn F. Silverman, M.D., M.P.H., one of the world's leading experts on the public health aspects of AIDS, frequently points out that, from the public's point of view, "the government said DDT was safe;

the government said toxic waste disposal systems were safe; the government said Three Mile Island was safe. Why should we expect people to believe the government now about AIDS?" A distrustful public has been unwilling to accept assurances that the medical facts about transmission of the AIDS virus are clear and settled. Conspiracy and cover-up theories still abound. Skeptics simply refuse to believe what they have been told, no matter how much evidence has been presented.

The prestigious National Academy of Sciences summed up the socio-political aspects of AIDS in a 1986 report to the nation:

> If a panel of public health experts, lawyers, economists and sociologists had been asked a decade ago to imagine a public health problem that would encompass the most difficult policy issues of the day, they could not have done better than to predict the appearance of AIDS.
>
> AIDS is the most complex public health challenge confronting modern medicine.
>
> . . . AIDS affects everybody, not just those who adhere to a particular lifestyle or who live in a certain part of the country. Government officials at all levels, business leaders, educators, health care professionals and everyone else who cares about how our society balances the needs of the community against those of individuals should participate in the development of reasonable and equitable approaches to the AIDS crisis.*

Writing in 1986 for the Washington Business Group on Health's publication, *Business and Health*, medical ethicists Ronald Bayer and Gerald Oppenheimer predicted that

> . . . living with the presence of AIDS will test the moral fiber of the nation. This is the social challenge of AIDS. Will it be met with compassion or anger? Will those who are ill and/or carry the virus be treated with

---

*Institute of Medicine, National Academy of Sciences, *Mobilizing Against AIDS, The Unfinished Story of a Virus*. Cambridge, Mass.: Harvard University Press, 1986.

dignity, or as pariahs, stripped of privacy and the right to function as
members of the community? Finally, will reason rule, or will the country
be swept along in a hysteria that encourages policies in both the private
and public sectors that are cruel and ineffective? How these questions
are answered will affect dimensions of social life extending far beyond
those immediately touched by AIDS.*

The public health establishment in this country and throughout
the world was ill-prepared in the 1970s and 1980s for a major
epidemic of any kind, having come to believe—as did the general
public—that large-scale infectious diseases were a thing of the past.
At the time the AIDS virus first invaded our society, public health
departments were staffed by a generation of scientists, physicians
and educators who, by and large, had never personally experienced
a major epidemic in the United States. They too were caught by
surprise.

AIDS Enters the Workplace

Even less prepared to cope with the complexities of a controversial
epidemic of disease have been the managers who are called upon
to deal with the consequences of AIDS in the workplace. Yet
managers in a variety of organizations were among the first policy
makers required to make decisions about managing this disease.
When the first cases of AIDS were diagnosed among employees
in the early 1980s, a great deal of mystery still surrounded the
cause of AIDS and the means by which a person could become
exposed to the disease. Human relations managers and corporate
attorneys suddenly found themselves in the arcane world of
epidemiology, consulting with scientists about obscure medical

*Ronald Bayer and Gerald Oppenheimer, "AIDS in the Workplace: The Ethical
Ramifications." *Business and Health*, Washington Business Group on Health,
January/February 1986, p. 30.

issues and struggling to arrive at rational corporate policies in the face of a great deal of uncertainty.

To the extent corporate America has responded at all to the tough issues surrounding AIDS, it has, by and large, responded with considerable clarity, compassion and rationality. The problem is that most organizations have not made a response, presumably in the hope that the issue would go away or affect only other organizations or perhaps would be easier to deal with tomorrow than it is today. Too many organizations simply have not prepared for the consequence of a case—or many cases—of AIDS among their workforce, and many of these organizations will regret their unpreparedness.

Successful management of. the consequences of the AIDS epidemic over the next decade will be an ongoing challenge, not only for the public health establishment, but for the managements of businesses, government agencies, nonprofit organizations, educational institutions, law enforcement agencies and health care establishments. AIDS has become, and will increasingly be, a significant management issue affecting organizations of all types and sizes and in all parts of the world. The epidemic and the issues it raises will continue to test the essential skills and wisdom of management at all levels. Fortunately, the pioneers in many of the organizations first affected by the epidemic in its earliest days have by now demonstrated that AIDS *is* manageable in the workplace. They have shown that certain approaches have a high probability of success, while others, a high probability of failure.

As a disease, AIDS has an unusually long "incubation period," the length of time between initial entry of the virus into the body and the development of identifiable symptoms of disease. Because of the long incubation period—at least three years and perhaps as long as ten years—the number of people infected with the virus but who are still seemingly healthy exceeds the number of people whose health has been damaged by the virus to the point where an AIDS diagnosis is possible. The long incubation period means that most of the cases of AIDS have not yet been discovered.

The Public Health Service and the CDC have estimated that, in the United States, there may be as many as forty people infected by the AIDS virus for *each* person diagnosed with AIDS. In other words, for each person who has reached the point of diagnosis, as many as forty may still be incubating the disease without symptoms having yet appeared. Therefore, the epidemic has the *probability* of becoming forty times worse than it appears to be at any given point in time. Based on existing rates of infection, then, and even without any further spread of the disease, for every organization thus far impacted by AIDS, at least forty other organizations are at high risk of encountering one or more cases in the next few years. The visible part of the AIDS epidemic—the reported diagnoses of AIDS—represents only the "tip of the iceberg."

By 1988, thousands of organizations in the U.S. and elsewhere in the world have already experienced the consequences of diagnosed AIDS within their workforce. Some of these organizations have handled the issue calmly, rationally and with minimum negative consequences to the organization or to the individuals involved. Companies like Westinghouse, Wells Fargo Bank, Trans-America, Bank of America, Levi Strauss, Digital Equipment Co., Dayton-Hudson, Chevron, Pacific Bell, Syntex and AT&T are role models for the rest of the nation. Still others have found themselves trapped in a horrendous and expensive quagmire of political, emotional, financial and legal issues.

Since AIDS tends to strike people in their economically most productive years, from twenty-five to forty-five, the people most likely to be diagnosed with AIDS in the future are generally employed somewhere in the workplace. Contrary to popular misconceptions, it is impossible to look at someone and identify that person as being at risk for AIDS; it is also impossible to diagnose a case of AIDS in advance.

AIDS has tended to strike people in certain recognizable "risk groups," and it is tempting to some people to think that the "typical" American workforce is not likely to contain anyone who belongs to one of those groups. To the contrary, what is more unlikely is that any workforce in America would consist entirely and exclusively of people in long-term monogamous relationships, people who for the past decade have had without exception only one sex partner, people who have *never* experimented with intravenous drugs, people who have *never* in the past decade had even one homosexual experience. It is just as unlikely that there exists a workforce in which no one is a hemophiliac or the sex partner of a hemophiliac, or that none of the workers have had a blood transfusion or have had sex with someone who has had a blood transfusion. Such a "pure" workforce denies the reality of contemporary American life.

If more than one-quarter of a million Americans will have developed AIDS by 1991, and many more will begin to suffer from AIDS-Related Complex within the same time frame, a great many organizations in this country will be touched by AIDS. While many organizations will manage to escape the effects of AIDS in the workplace through sheer statistical luck, no organization will be exempt from its consequences; and all organizations should be prepared to deal with AIDS as it appears in the workplace in various forms. In his report to the nation on AIDS, the Surgeon General of the United States put it very simply: ". . . work sites should have a plan in operation for education of the workforce and accommodation of AIDS or ARC patients before the first such case appears at the work site."

In 1987, two noted epidemiologists, Donald Francis, M.D., and James Chin, M.D., prepared for the *Journal of the American Medical Association* a master plan for controlling the AIDS epidemic. Their plan included asking employers to become involved in planning for AIDS:

The impact of AIDS on the private sector is large and growing. The direct medical costs, the benefit support costs and the general social upheaval (due primarily to unfounded concerns about the possibility of casual-contact transmission) will continue to take a major toll within the business community. Much of this toll is preventable, including that related to unfounded fears of infection.*

The AIDS epidemic has already touched a great many organizations. Some were prepared for it and handled the issues well; others were not prepared and made significant and costly mistakes. Based on the experience of businesses that have been forced to cope with the consequence of AIDS in the workplace, advance preparation following a calm and objective analysis of the issues is the fundamental difference between success and failure in managing AIDS, just as it is with any other workplace issue.

Consider these workplace scenarios, several of which could apply to your own organization:

- You are a department manager with more than 100 employees. An employee comes to you in confidence, nervously explaining that he has been diagnosed with AIDS. He wants to know what your organization will do about medical and disability benefits, and he is concerned about his continued employment. He wants to work as long as he can, and he doesn't want anyone else in the organization to know about his condition. What will you say, and to whom? What will you do?

- You are the chief executive of a sizable company. Your organization has not yet encountered AIDS, but you recognize the challenge it poses from what you read in the business press. Should you have a policy about AIDS? What should it be? How can you best go about determining an organizational policy towards AIDS? Who needs to participate in setting the policy?

---

*Donald P. Francis, M.D., D.Sc., and James Chin, M.D., M.P.H., "The Prevention of Acquired Immunodeficiency Syndrome in the United States, An Objective Strategy for Medicine, Public Health, Business and the Community." *Journal of the American Medical Association*, March 13, 1987, p. 1357.

What are other organizations doing? What does the law require? Are there actions you can take now to avoid or minimize the cost of this disease?

- You are a union representative. The company has asked you to participate in a discussion on what approach to take if an employee is diagnosed with AIDS. What position will you take on behalf of your union and its members? You will have to consider the two major aspects of the union's role and responsibility—protecting the jobs of ill or disabled employees *and* ensuring the safety of co-workers on the job. You suspect that many of your union members may not want a person with AIDS to be on the job. How will you approach the company on this issue?

- You are a human relations manager. You receive a panicky call from a department head. Rumors are spreading that an employee in the department has AIDS. Co-workers are extremely upset about the possibility of becoming infected, and a delegation has just advised the supervisor that they will not return to work tomorrow if the person suspected of having AIDS is still on the job. Two of the employees within the department are pregnant; the father of one of them is a labor lawyer. How will you advise the supervisor?

- You are a supervisor. A long-time employee has confided in you that the person with whom she shares a work station is probably gay. Although she has never said anything about it before, she is now concerned about becoming exposed to AIDS, and she wants a change of work partner, or a transfer to another work assignment. Both are excellent employees, and you do not want to lose them. How will you handle this situation?

- You are a benefits manager. When he returned from a seminar about "new management issues for the coming decade," your CEO requested from you an immediate estimate of the potential cost to your company of the AIDS epidemic and an actionable plan for avoiding the cost. What will you report?

▪ You are an employee assistance counselor. A worried mother of a teenage boy asks for assistance in getting AIDS prevention information for her son, who now has a summer job with your company. She thinks he may be shooting drugs. How will you advise her? For that matter, what are you going to do or say about AIDS and sex and drugs to your own teenage children?

▪ You are a supervisor. One of your employees, who you suspect has used drugs from time to time, is increasingly absent due to illness, and his work performance is slipping. You wonder if he may have contracted AIDS from sharing drug needles or from having sex with his drug-user girlfriend. You have no proof of either. Can you demand a medical examination?

▪ You are a computer center manager. A female employee is known to associate after work with a sexually active crowd of young people. What will you do if a fellow employee raises the issue of her possible exposure to AIDS? Are the other workers safe, sharing the equipment she uses? Are there precautions the department should take?

▪ You are an in-house company nurse. A female employee comes to you because she and her new husband want to have a child. She has a sexually active past and is concerned that she could have been exposed to the AIDS virus at some point before her marriage. She's reluctant to discuss the issue with her husband. Should she take the AIDS antibody test? What advice will you give her? If you are able to perform the test at work, what will you do if her test is positive? Who will you have to tell about the test result?

▪ You are a food service department manager. One of the cooks in the company cafeteria is losing weight and looks sick. Although he has been "clean" for the three years he's been with your department, he has a history of IV drug use before being hired by your organization. If he was exposed to AIDS during his drug-use period, could he now be infecting the entire organization through the food in the cafeteria? Should you demand a medical examination? How would you handle employee panic if your concerns become common knowledge?

- You are the chief administrator of a private school. What will you do if one of your teachers contracts AIDS and wants to continue working? Or if one of your students is diagnosed HIV-positive, and his parents demand that he stay in school?

- You are responsible for safety within your organization. You also conduct First Aid and CPR courses, in which you train employees to go to the aid of co-workers in the event of a factory accident. What about exposing people to blood during an accident? Should you modify your training and safety programs because of potential AIDS risk?

- You are a supervisor of a company security department. Your employees are becoming increasingly nervous about exposure to AIDS. They must protect company property from burglars and shoplifters who they say are frequently IV drug-users, and IV drug-users are also likely carriers of the AIDS virus. They cite newspaper reports of police officers wearing gloves even during AIDS-related political demonstrations. They want to wear gloves even when on plainclothes undercover assignment, although to do so would certainly "blow their cover" and render them virtually useless for the intended purpose. What do you do about the issue?

- You manage a telephone switchboard for a large governmental agency. There are several shifts each day, and everyone shares the same equipment. Your agency does not have a policy about AIDS one way or another; it usually does not address new issues until much later than do other organizations. So it is unlikely that a policy statement on AIDS will be forthcoming. Suppose the issue of AIDS comes up in your department? How are you going to handle it, considering that, with little help from your supervisor, you will likely be blamed by management if a crisis over AIDS erupts in your department. How can you protect yourself and maintain the effectiveness of your department?

None of these is a hypothetical situation. Each has been faced by a real manager in a real organization. These scenarios represent only a few of the issues that have arisen and will continue to come up about AIDS in the workplace environment. Some of the issues are relatively simple; others are quite complex. In some of the examples, the issues were handled calmly, with courage and conviction and an understanding of the facts. In others the issues were so mishandled that it led to an embarrassing nightmare of disruption, litigation and loss of time, money and productivity.

The issue in each of these situations represents a potential disaster both for the organization and for the manager responsible for taking action. Conversely, each of these scenarios can be handled effectively. Each situation can be dealt with in a manner consistent with existing company policies, in compliance with the law and in a way that employees and stockholders will recognize as rational, fair and responsible.

2 ‖ Understanding AIDS: The Epidemic, the Virus and the Disease

In order for managers to understand the relationship of AIDS to the workplace and to develop appropriate policies within the organizational setting, they first must understand AIDS itself—AIDS as a virus that causes disease, AIDS as a disease that operates within the human body to destroy the immune system, and AIDS as an epidemic that is taking a certain path through the population. A great deal of information is available about each of these aspects of AIDS. There is, however, also the need to understand AIDS as a socio-political and cultural phenomenon of our time. There is less certainty about the socio-political factors, which, of course, depend on the beliefs and behavior of people and not on the more predictable behavior of viruses.

For every question that one might have about the cause and the epidemiology of AIDS, the response must necessarily contain both "good news and bad news." The bad news is that there *never* can be undebatable certainty about any medical condition that afflicts the human body. In spite of the startling progress of medical and scientific research in the twentieth century, much that transpires within the human body remains a mystery. It seems that for every additional piece of knowledge we acquire about human physiology and disease, new questions are raised. To complicate matters, our understanding of disease transmission depends in large part on the willingness of people to tell the truth about how they might have been exposed to the disease. In the case of a disease transmitted through socially stigmatized practices, there is a great temptation to deny the circumstances of exposure. Thus it is difficult ever to be completely certain about all aspects of a disease and its effect on the human body, and AIDS is no exception.

To make matters worse, doctors and medical researchers generally refuse to speak about disease in terms of certainty. Physicians are trained to speak only in terms of "medical probabilities," not medical certainties. As a consequence, scientists and public health officials are trained to say *"there is no evidence"* that such-and-such exists, rather than "it has never happened" or "it won't happen."

When people hear "there is no evidence," especially in answer to a question about the more remote means of AIDS transmission, they mistakenly assume that there is a hidden message in the choice of words, and that the doctor is really saying "there is no evidence, but some evidence could turn up later." Unfortunately, for most people, the words seem to mean "we don't know" or "maybe." For example, if scientists were asked whether it would be possible to contract cancer from reading this book, most would respond, "There is no evidence that reading this book can cause cancer." Fewer scientists would be willing to make the statement, "No, it's impossible to get cancer from reading this book." The expression "there is no evidence" is an instilled characteristic of scientific discussion and the public must learn to accept it for what it really means and not give it any more significance than it actually has.

The "good news" is that a great deal is now known about AIDS. After years of study in which tens of thousands of AIDS cases have been analyzed in a variety of settings and in a number of countries, this disease proves to be extremely predictable. There is considerable scientific agreement about its means of transmission. For several years now, there have been no surprises about the transmission of AIDS and none are likely to occur in the future. Every new piece of evidence tends to confirm existing conclusions about transmission, and demonstrates how difficult it is to transmit the AIDS virus from person to person. In view of this, there is ample, widely recognized, scientific evidence on which to base an organizational response to AIDS. Whether we like to admit it or not, thousands of policies affecting millions of employees about any number of issues are made in organizations every day on the basis of evidence that is much less concrete than the evidence we have on AIDS.

The Course of the Epidemic

AIDS is a blood-borne, sexually transmitted disease. Its methods of spreading from person to person are similar to the means by which other venereal diseases are transmitted, but quite different from the means of transmission of flu, colds and other classic epidemics.

The virus that causes AIDS—Human Immunodeficiency Virus —may not have existed prior to the 1960s. Its origin is unknown, and irrelevant to how society will deal with AIDS in the future or how organizations should deal with AIDS in the workplace. Nevertheless, because people usually want to know where something came from and how it began, we can postulate the most likely origins of the virus.

Scientists have traced the AIDS virus to countries of south central Africa, like Zaire and Uganda, Mali and Kenya, where it was present before 1970. It is not known whether the virus originated in Africa, or whether it came to Africa from somewhere else. We do know that in several countries of south central Africa, the AIDS virus has been found in stored blood supplies that date as far back as the 1960s.

Medical researchers have developed two theories to explain how and where the virus began. The popular theory is that it originated in animal populations—the green monkey is considered the prime candidate—and then was transmitted to human beings, perhaps changing its form somewhat in the process and becoming what we now know as the AIDS virus. Another, but less likely, theory is that the AIDS virus may have existed in humans in a slightly different and benign form for many years in that part of the world, and then for unknown reasons mutated into the form we now know as HIV. Viruses tend to mutate and to change their characteristics over long periods of time. Either the mutation theory or the animal origin theory could be correct. In any event, for whatever reason, humanity first began to encounter the virus during the 1960s and 1970s.

The medical consequences of the AIDS virus may have gone unnoticed in Africa for the first several years, in part because of the long incubation period of the disease, and in part because of the multitude of medical problems that already taxed the inadequate health care systems of those countries.

Exactly what path the virus took from Africa to Europe and the United States is not known. The large volume of commercial traffic moving among these countries presented ample opportunities for the virus to be carried in a variety of directions within a short period of time. The international air corridors are filled with jumbo jets carrying tourists, business people, airline personnel and others. The Boeing 747 provides an efficient means of transporting a new virus from continent to continent in a matter of a few hours.

It is now known from examining old stored blood supplies in the U.S. that the AIDS virus arrived in New York no later than 1977, and that it reached the West Coast cities of Los Angeles and San Francisco by 1978, quickly fanning out to other American urban centers, and from there to more remote and less densely populated areas. Within a decade, the AIDS virus was found in every state and in most cities and towns of America. By the 1980s, the virus had found its way through various routes to virtually every country in the world.

It is useful to understand the socio-cultural conditions that existed at the time the AIDS virus was introduced into American society and from which the course of the epidemic was derived. Sociological and cultural factors have a lot to do with how the virus was spread, with who tended to get the disease and with how the epidemic came to be identified only with certain groups.

It is ironic that the AIDS virus arrived in America at the very height of the so-called sexual liberation movement, which began during World War II, continued through the Korean War and Viet Nam era and reached a peak during the "sex, drugs and rock'n roll" period of the 1960s and 1970s. At no time were the mores of the sexual liberation movement practiced more vigorously than during the late 1970s among urban homosexual males, who enjoyed what was for them a degree of freedom and openness unparalleled in modern times. Like the heterosexual hippies of the 1960s, urban gay men in cities like New York, Los Angeles, Houston, San Francisco, Miami, Dallas, Chicago, Phoenix, Atlanta and Boston, began engaging in unlimited sexual interactions. For many of these young men, life took on the characteristics of an ongoing party, complete with popular institutions like bathhouses that facilitated free and easy sexual encounters among large numbers of people. Syphilis, gonorrhea and other sexually transmitted diseases were easily cured by a single shot of antibiotics with no significant side- or after-effects. For a generation of gay men who had reached adulthood after the abolition of venereal disease as a medical threat, "recreational sex," as it was known, became a popular pastime, practiced by tens of thousands on an international scale with seemingly no negative consequences in sight.

By 1982 when the first diagnoses of AIDS began to appear among gay men, large numbers of them had already been infected with the AIDS virus and were incubating the disease. By the time AIDS was shown to be caused by a sexually transmitted virus, opportunities for prevention among a large population of urban homosexual men had already been lost.

Data on rates of infection among homosexual men is scarce. In San Francisco, the city for which accurate data on homosexual and bisexual men is most readily available, nearly one-half of gay men in that city became infected with the AIDS virus before it was even identified. Health Department studies there estimated that out of a total population of 675,000 citizens, up to 35,000 men were infected and incubating the virus. Effective AIDS prevention programs were able to halt new infections by the virus, once there was clarity about the cause and prevention of AIDS, but by then, the die was cast for many in that community. Comparable rates of infection could be found in the gay communities of most major American and European cities.

Homosexual men not only provided the first-diagnosed cases of AIDS, but constituted such an enormous pool of infected people from which other cases would be diagnosed, that the future course of the AIDS epidemic would be statistically obscured by this significantly skewed data. Just as Legionnaire's disease became identified with the members of the American Legion who were first diagnosed with that disease, AIDS became identified in the public mind with homosexual and bisexual men.

Almost simultaneously with the entry of the virus into the gay community, the AIDS virus also quickly found its way into the populations of people who use illegal intravenous drugs, especially in New York, New Jersey and South Florida. The profile of this population was generally quite different from that of infected homosexual men. Intravenous drug-users tended to be heterosexual males or females, nonwhite, uneducated, poor and unemployed.

Comparable to the disease-spreading opportunities in the bathhouses of the gay community are the "shooting galleries" of IV drug-users, places where people meet to purchase and use illegal drugs. Heroin and cocaine are more readily available in "shooting galleries" than are the needles for injecting the drugs. As a consequence, a single needle is passed around and used by dozens, if not hundreds of people, without any attempt at sterilization.

Even outside the "shooting galleries," drug-users tend to socialize for the purpose of sharing drugs. Cultural traditions among users call for the passing around of a single needle to be shared by all those present. Needles for injecting drugs are available in the U.S. only by prescription, and are in short supply among users; thus sharing needles has become a necessity for drug-users as well as a social convention. The practice of sharing needles could not have been more ideal for transmitting a blood-borne disease to large numbers of people very quickly.

Within a few years, tens of thousands of IV drug-users were infected by the virus and quickly became the second largest "risk group" for AIDS. They also served as the path for AIDS to reach the population of multiple-partner heterosexuals, especially in the Black and Hispanic communities. Consequently, they became the source of AIDS among newborn infants; by 1988 the virus had affected one out of every sixty-one babies born in New York state.

The unique conditions that existed in both the gay community and the population of intravenous drug-users during the first decade after the entry of the AIDS virus were ideal for quickly infecting large numbers of people, and for doing so before the "early warning signs" of the epidemic had appeared. AIDS cases were diagnosed so overwhelmingly from those two communities for the first several years that the public believed that this new disease would be contained within those two communities. AIDS became so identified in the public mind with homosexuals and IV drug-users, two groups which had little public support, that the fact of this identification has colored official response to the epidemic, in both the public and the private sector.

The early heavily skewed statistics tended to obscure the fact that as a sexually transmitted disease, AIDS could be transmitted without regard to sexual orientation, and would ultimately put heterosexuals at risk if they had multiple sexual partners. The principal difference for heterosexuals would be the lower statistical odds of having sex with an infected non–drug-using opposite-gender partner. The odds for heterosexuals were still substantially lower than the odds of a homosexual encountering an infected homosexual for sex, or of an IV drug-user sharing a needle with an infected drug-using carrier of the virus.

During the early days of the AIDS epidemic hemophiliacs and recipients of blood transfusions also became infected with the virus through their medical dependence on blood and blood products. These two groups of people became infected between 1977, when the AIDS virus arrived in this country, and the spring of 1985, when blood screening programs were put into effect.

Large numbers of hemophiliacs were infected by the AIDS virus between 1977 and 1985. Of the hemophiliacs in the U.S., about 90 percent of those tested were infected with the AIDS virus before Factor VIII, the blood-clotting substance, was made safe. For reasons that aren't yet clear, despite the high rate of infection among hemophiliacs, not many of them have actually been diagnosed with AIDS. It could be that the incubation period for the disease might be longer for those having this particular medical condition, or it's possible that something about the manufacturing process for the Factor VIII clotting material might have weakened the virus. While the ultimate outcome for AIDS in the hemophiliac population isn't yet known, it is clear that the majority of American hemophiliacs carry the AIDS antibody and presumably are able to sexually pass the virus on to their wives or sexual partners.

The other category of people infected during the early days of the epidemic were those individuals who received transfusions of infected blood between 1977 and 1985, when the blood screening programs were placed in operation at the blood banks. During the first six years of diagnosed cases of AIDS, about 2 percent of the total cases were contracted through contaminated blood transfusions. Since all blood is now screened for the presence of the AIDS antibody and is discarded if it is suspected of infection, the blood supply is safer than it has ever been. Nevertheless, because of the long incubation period for this disease, we can expect to see additional cases of AIDS diagnosed in the future as a result of pre-1985 blood transfusions.

The Virus

AIDS is a condition caused by a virus with several interesting characteristics that literally shape the nature of this epidemic. The first characteristic of the virus to understand is that, outside of the human body, out in the environment, in the air, on environmental surfaces, or even on human skin, this virus is unusually fragile and harmless.

The HIV is a weak microorganism that requires a moist, temperature-controlled environment in which to survive. It does not live well outside the body. Sunlight kills this virus. Common household cleaning products such as Lysol or diluted Clorox or even plain soap and water kill the virus. The hot water in a home or restaurant dishwasher easily kills the virus. The virus cannot live for very long on environmental surfaces, and even if it did, it would remain harmless without a way to enter into the human bloodstream via the mucous membranes that are found within someone's body.

This virus does not even have the necessary built-in genetic mechanism—the genetic code—to reproduce itself. To achieve reproduction, the AIDS virus requires an elaborate process that takes place only inside the human body, and which requires the use of genetic material borrowed from the human body.

If you were to put a single bacterium on an environmental surface, and if the conditions were right, that single bacterium would begin to reproduce. Over time, there might soon be thousands or even millions of bacteria living on that surface, derived from a single original cell. By contrast, if you put a single

AIDS virus on an environmental surface, even if the conditions were superb and the virus managed to live, there would never be more than a single AIDS virus on the surface. Out in an open environment, the AIDS virus is incapable of reproduction. Out in an open environment, the AIDS virus is incapable of harming human beings.

On the other hand, if the virus penetrates *into* the human body and enters *into* the human bloodstream, then it is capable of crippling the very immune system that protects us from disease. Inside the body, the virus is powerful and can be extremely damaging to human health. We are extremely fortunate that such a devastating virus is so difficult to effectively transmit from person to person.

The AIDS Virus in the Body

Inside the human bloodstream, this virus has the capability of identifying and attaching itself to a specific white blood cell known as a "T-Helper Cell Lymphocyte." This particular kind of lymphocyte is a component of the immune system; it has a major role in managing the response of the immune system whenever the human body is invaded by a disease. The function of these lymphocytes is only just now being understood. T-Helper Cell Lymphocytes help turn on and manage the immune response; their existence is essential to our health. There are millions of these T-Helper Cell Lymphocytes in our bodies, as well as other types of lymphocytes, each with a specialized function.

Once inside the circulatory system, the AIDS virus becomes one more part of the enormously extensive network of rivers we call the bloodstream. The virus has no independent means of propulsion and cannot control its own motion. It simply floats along with billions of other cells through miles of veins, arteries and capillaries. On the surface of the virus, however, are "hooks," called "antigens," which allow the virus to attach itself to other cells that have "receptors"—something like docking ports—that effectively match the design of the antigen. The antigens of the AIDS virus are a perfect match for the receptors on the surfaces of the T-Helper Cell Lymphocytes in the bloodstream. Consequently, if the virus encounters a T-Helper Cell Lymphocyte during its journey down the bloodstream, it can attach itself to the lymphocyte's receptors. The virus can literally bind itself to the surface of the lymphocyte, which is a much larger cell than the virus itself.

Once the virus attaches to the lymphocyte, it is capable of injecting its genetic material, its ribonucleic acid, or RNA, into the lymphocyte's DNA—the human DNA. The virus is able to actually "pirate" the T-cell's genetic machinery, turning the lymphocyte into a factory for making AIDS viruses. The virus cannot reproduce by itself, but it can take control of the lymphocyte's genetic processes through the use of an enzyme called "reverse transcriptase." Once the virus has taken control of the lymphocyte's reproductive processes, it can remain dormant for extensive periods of time or, at that time or much later, begin using the genetic material of the lymphocyte to produce hundreds and perhaps thousands of additional viruses. What factors determine whether the virus remains dormant or begins reproduction are still unknown.

In the latter case, if the reproduction process is stimulated, the newly created viruses each eventually break out of the lymphocyte's body and goes its own way attaching to other lymphocytes and repeating the process. As a consequence of all this reproduction, the "factory" lymphocytes in which the viruses are produced soon die.

Over time, usually over several years, more and more viruses are produced, and more and more lymphocytes are destroyed. The human body does not manufacture unlimited quantities of new lymphocytes. Lymphocytes are among the longest-living cells in the human body, and normally live for about twenty-five years. The body would not typically need to produce large numbers of these lymphocytes, and at some point in the process the supply of T-Helper Cell Lymphocytes available in the bloodstream reaches a critically low level, at which the immune system can no longer properly function. The body then begins to be attacked by "opportunistic diseases," diseases that are often present in our environment, but which do not harm people with fundamentally sound immune systems. Of the possible opportunistic diseases, the ones most commonly associated with AIDS are pneumocystis pneumonia, a lung disease caused by a protozoan, and a form of capillary cancer called Kaposi's sarcoma.

People with depressed immune systems also tend to experience major problems with infections caused by ordinary fungi. Fungi of various kinds are always present in the bodies of healthy people. Fungi are a normal part of our existence, and our immune systems routinely keep them in check. In people with AIDS, the fungi inside the body can simply grow out of control, causing a variety of annoying and sometimes serious medical problems.

The Long "Incubation Period" for AIDS

The elapsed time between the entry of the AIDS virus into the bloodstream and the point when the opportunistic diseases first appear after the damage to the immune system has reached a critical stage is called the "incubation period." The incubation period for AIDS is usually three to five years. In some people, the incubation period might even be as long as ten years. There is a great deal of individual variation in the incubation period for AIDS. We are all different; and our physical reactions to disease are often quite different. For any one of us, the incubation period might depend in part on our individual physiology, the status of our immune system at the time of original infection, the method of infection, the quantity of virus to which we were exposed and a variety of other physical and psychological co-factors.

During the incubation period and before the appearance of the opportunistic infections that signal the onset of AIDS, the person infected with the virus would have no physical indication that he or she carried the virus. Most of the one to two million Americans estimated by the CDC to be infected and incubating the disease have no knowledge that the virus is inside their bodies, slowly destroying their immune system. During this incubation period, infected persons can presumably pass the virus on to others either through unprotected sexual intercourse (sexual intercourse without the protection of a condom) or through direct contact between the bloodstream of an already-infected person and the bloodstream of the person being infected.

Transmission of the Virus

Transmission of the AIDS virus from person to person requires that the virus (1) be able to leave the bloodstream of one person in whom the virus is present; and (2) remain safely within a moist and temperature-controlled environment long enough to (3) enter the body of another person through the internal mucous membranes, and to do so in sufficient quantity to cause infection.

Unlike the virus that causes the flu, the AIDS virus cannot be transmitted through the air. It has never been transmitted through sneezing or coughing. If it were at all possible for the disease to be transmitted through the air, by breathing or sneezing or coughing, then by now, after more than a decade, someone would have contracted the virus from simply being in the same room with a person who is a carrier. AIDS is not transmitted that way, and the many studies of household living arrangements have demonstrated that AIDS is not spread by what is called "casual contact."

The ways in which the AIDS virus *has* been transmitted from person to person have been studied in great detail since the first cases of AIDS were reported. Transmission has always been the burning issue for scientists interested in studying this epidemic. Any researcher who discovers a new way in which AIDS can be transmitted is guaranteed a featured speaking opportunity at the next international AIDS conference, front-page coverage in most newspapers, and opportunities to publish articles in scientific journals. Yet epidemiologists in many countries have independently evaluated possible methods of transmission and have reached the same conclusions. Within the inherent limits of medical certainty, the methods of AIDS transmission are definite, specific and, fortunately, very limited. AIDS is difficult to catch.

AIDS can be transmitted from one person to another by three transmission methods. The most common method is through *sexual intercourse*. The second method is through *direct blood-to-blood contact*, between the bloodstream of one person and the bloodstream of another person. The third method is maternal transmission between an infected and pregnant woman and her unborn child. All cases of transmission of the AIDS virus ever studied fit into one of these three categories. No other methods have ever been found anywhere in any country during the entire course of the AIDS epidemic. The three methods by which AIDS has been transmitted—unprotected sexual intercourse, mother-to-child transmission, and direct blood-to-blood contact—can be further subdivided for greater understanding.

The largest number of AIDS cases in this country and around the world have been transmitted by sexual intercourse. For this reason, AIDS should be classified as a "venereal or sexually transmitted disease (STD)." The AIDS virus can be transmitted sexually because lymphocytes, the white blood cells in which the AIDS virus reproduces within the human body, can be found in substantial quantities in semen and vaginal fluids. When the infected lymphocytes find their way into the semen or vaginal fluids, the AIDS virus goes with them. Sexual intercourse is an excellent way in which to transmit the virus directly from one person to another, via fluid in a moist, temperature-controlled environment, out of the body of one person and directly into the interior of the body of another. AIDS can be transmitted sexually if there are infected lymphocytes in the semen or vaginal fluids of one sex partner, and if those infected lymphocytes are allowed to contact the mucous membranes inside the body of the uninfected partner.

In the case of homosexual males, the AIDS virus has been most commonly transmitted through anal intercourse, an especially effective means of transmitting the virus. During anal intercourse, large quantities of semen containing the virus-infected lymphocytes are injected into the fragile tissues of an area of the body with few immunological defense mechanisms. The vagina and the mouth have substantial defensive systems that tend to fend off disease. Nevertheless, AIDS, like other sexually transmitted diseases, can be transmitted vaginally or orally, as well as anally. Oral transmission is the least effective method, because the enzymes and digestive acids of the mouth and stomach tend to kill the virus.

Sexual transmission of the AIDS virus works heterosexually as well as homosexually, and the virus can be passed from women to men and from men to women. A study of the heterosexual partners of virus-infected men and women conducted at the University of California indicates that unprotected vaginal intercourse does not always transmit the virus to the uninfected partner. A study of the case of an African businessman who had sex with twenty female partners, without using condoms, over the course of several months before realizing that he was infected with AIDS found that twelve of the women became infected by the virus, but eight did not. AIDS appears to be difficult to transmit even under ideal circumstances.

Condoms have been found to be a generally effective barrier against the AIDS virus. Studies conducted at the University of California Medical School proved that if the condom is used correctly, the AIDS virus cannot penetrate the condom material. The impenetrability of the condom material is higher with latex condoms than with the so-called natural condoms made of lambskin, although it should be remembered that condoms are not necessarily foolproof in actual use.

Within the transmission category of "blood-to-blood contact," only three subcategories of transmission have ever been found among the tens of thousands of cases studied. Each of these subcategories is a variation on the same theme.

The first subcategory is that of *sharing IV drug needles* which accounts for nearly 20 percent of all cases of AIDS in America. Transmission by sharing unsterilized needles is easy to understand. If you were to inject drugs into your vein with a needle and then hand the same needle to someone else to use, whatever came into contact with the needle while it was in your bloodstream could be injected directly into the vein of the other person. This would constitute direct contact between the bloodstreams of the two people.

Proper sterilization of the needle between uses would kill the virus, although drug-users frequently lack either the knowledge or the patience required for the sterilization of their drug apparatus. Recent attempts to persuade IV drug-users to clean their needles with bleach have met with some success. Ordinary chlorine bleach kills the virus on contact and can be used to sterilize needles between uses.

The second subcategory of blood-to-blood contact is transmission by *receipt of contaminated blood transfusions or of contaminated blood products*. Included are hemophiliac recipients of contaminated Factor VIII clotting medication made from unscreened blood supplies before 1985. Again, it is easy to understand how transfusion of contaminated blood, or the injection into the body of blood clotting medication made from contaminated blood could spread the virus. The virus lives and reproduces within the bloodstream. So if virus-contaminated blood is taken from one person's body and then injected or transfused into someone else's body, the virus is carried in the blood and is able to reproduce within the body of the recipient. This category of AIDS transmission should no longer represent a threat since blood and blood products are now screened in the U.S. and Western countries. If antibodies to the

AIDS virus are identified in a unit of blood, the blood is discarded and not used.

The third subcategory of blood-to-blood contact is extremely rare, but does involve workplace exposure within certain health care professions where *occupational contact with blood* is common. A handful of health care workers have been infected by the virus, either through accidentally sticking themselves with needles used on AIDS patients, or by allowing their cut or severely chapped hands to come in contact with large quantities of patient blood, without the protection of gloves and in violation of standard infection control procedures for health care workers. Considering how many thousands of health care workers deal directly with AIDS patients in hospitals and doctors' offices all over the world, including the many doctors and nurses who worked with AIDS patients during the several years before AIDS was known to be a communicable disease, the number of health care workers infected in this way is astonishingly small, demonstrating once again that AIDS is an extraordinarily difficult disease to transmit accidentally.

If a woman becomes infected with the AIDS virus through one of the other means of transmission (sexual intercourse, the sharing of IV needles, or through a blood transfusion), and then becomes pregnant, there is a 50/50 chance that the child will become infected with the virus from the mother's blood at some point before or during birth. *Maternal transmission* is a consequence of transmission by one of the other direct methods—sexual intercourse or blood contact. Maternal transmission is becoming a major problem as increasing numbers of newborn babies enter the world already infected with the AIDS virus. In 1988, the virus had infected one out of every sixty-one babies born in New York State.

In the ten years since the beginning of this epidemic no one has ever found a method of transmission for the AIDS virus that does not fall within the methods described above. There has not been a single exception. In addition, the theoretical understanding of the AIDS virus and its operating characteristics is totally consistent with these methods. As you can see, each of these methods requires the most intimate kind of contact, and in fact requires some degree of conscious and deliberate interaction between two people. AIDS transmission requires virtually direct injection of the virus into a person's body. AIDS is properly called a "disease of consenting adults," because, except for nonconsenting acts like rape based on violence, no one can infect you with the AIDS virus without some conscious and deliberate act on your part.

In the same way that we know how a person can become infected, we also know how a person cannot get the virus. You cannot get AIDS from simply being in the same room with someone who has AIDS. You cannot get AIDS by shaking hands with someone, or by sharing a friendly hug. You can't get AIDS by working alongside of, or by sharing work equipment with, a co-worker who has AIDS. You can't get AIDS from food or beverages served in a restaurant, any more than you could get syphilis or gonorrhea from food or beverages served in a restaurant. You can't get AIDS from a hottub, unless you have sex in one. You cannot get AIDS from a telephone or computer keyboard. You can't get AIDS from a swimming pool. You can't get AIDS from mosquitos or other insects. You can't get AIDS by riding in an airplane or otherwise using public transportation. You can't get AIDS by touching a person with AIDS or by visiting an AIDS patient in a hospital or in his or her home.

Specifically, insofar as the conventional workplace is concerned, "you *cannot* get AIDS from a co-worker at work, except by doing something at work that you are not being paid to do!" AIDS is not transmissible between co-workers in the ordinary workplace environment. Persons with AIDS are not a threat to co-workers or to the public.

Given the well-established means by which AIDS can be transmitted, the Centers for Disease Control and the United States Public Health Service issued formal guidelines in 1985 for AIDS in the Workplace. These guidelines are still in effect and have since been confirmed by the Surgeon General, the National Academy of Sciences, the American Medical Association, various independent research scientists, and a myriad of American corporations and institutions. The CDC Guidelines for AIDS in the Workplace, include the following clear statements:

> . . . AIDS is a bloodborne, sexually-transmitted disease that is not spread by casual contact.

> No known risk of transmission to coworkers, clients or consumers exists from [AIDS-] infected workers in . . . offices, schools, factories [or] construction sites.

> . . . casual contact with saliva and tears does not result in transmission of infection.

> The kind of nonsexual person-to-person contact that generally occurs among workers and clients or consumers in the workplace does not pose a risk for transmission [of the AIDS virus].

> AIDS is not transmitted through preparation of food or beverages . . .

> . . . Food service workers known to be infected with AIDS should not be restricted from work unless they have another infection or illness for which such restriction should be warranted.

> Workers known to be infected with [AIDS] should not be restricted from work solely based on this finding. Moreover, they should not be restricted from using telephones, office equipment, toilets, showers, eating facilities and water fountains. *

The National Academy of Science's Institute of Medicine points

---

*Centers for Disease Control, United States Public Health Service, "PHS Recommendations for Preventing Transmission of Infection with HTLV-3/LAV in the Workplace." *Morbidity and Mortality Weekly Report 34* (45) (November 15, 1985), pp. 681–695.

out that ". . . the virus that causes AIDS does not penetrate the skin, the . . . cells lining the respiratory tract, or the mucosa of the digestive tract. Thus, the disease cannot be transmitted by a handshake, by a cough or sneeze, or by the consumption of food prepared by someone with AIDS. Moderate heat, . . . standard solutions of almost all common disinfectants, and an ordinary dilution of household bleach . . . inactivate [the AIDS virus]."

Further, "long-term studies of the families of adult and pediatric AIDS patients and of thousands of health care personnel demonstrate that the virus is not transmitted by any daily activity related to living with or caring for an AIDS patient. Siblings of children with AIDS have remained free of infection even after sharing beds and toothbrushes with a sick child."

On the subject of casual contact, the Institute noted that "fears about the possibility of catching AIDS through casual contact were most intense among the general public shortly after researchers announced that they could isolate the virus from body fluids other than blood and semen. Subsequent studies have shown, however, that the virus is very rare in secretions such as tears and saliva, and even when it is present, the levels are probably too low to play a role in infection. . . . The likelihood of infection appears to depend in part on the quantity of virus transmitted; a small dose probably cannot withstand normal body defense mechanisms. This would explain the rarity of infection among health care workers who accidentally stick themselves with infected needles."*

The press's use of the term "the sharing of body fluids" has been an unfortunate and misleading choice of language. The body fluids of concern for AIDS transmission are (1) blood, (2) semen, and (3) vaginal fluids. The more general phrase "the sharing of body

---

*Institute of Medicine, National Academy of Sciences, *Mobilizing Against AIDS, The Unfinished Story of a Virus*. Cambridge, Mass.: Harvard University Press, 1986, pp. 10–11.

fluids" used by the media was originally a euphemism designed to allow reporters to avoid references to semen and vaginal fluids in "family newspapers." According to Dr. Jay Levy, a pioneering AIDS researcher who has specifically studied the issue of body fluids, to infect someone with AIDS from saliva or tears, "you would need at least a quart of saliva or a quart of tears, and then you'd need to introduce these body fluids directly into the bloodstream to cause infection."*

In short, because the AIDS virus is transmitted from person to person only by sexual intercourse or by an activity requiring direct contact between the bloodstream of one person and the bloodstream of another, the AIDS virus cannot be transmitted between co-workers in the ordinary course of business activity. Under those circumstances, there is *no* scientific basis for concern about AIDS transmission from employee to employee in the workplace based on legitimate work activities.

It necessarily follows that there is no legitimate medical or scientific reason to treat AIDS in the workplace differently than any other significant life-threatening illness. Employee fears about AIDS can be seen as resulting from ignorance or bias and can be dealt with calmly through educational programs or counseling. If you are concerned about how to respond to employees' concerns that AIDS might be a threat to them at work, ask yourself how you would react if an employee were concerned about catching leukemia from a co-worker? Or if co-workers refused to work with someone who had a heart attack, based on fears that they might contract heart disease, how would you handle that situation? Just because AIDS is a relatively new disease does not mean that

---

*Jay Levy, M.D., interviewed in the videotape, "An Epidemic of Fear: AIDS in the Workplace." Produced in cooperation with the Business Leadership Task Force of the Bay Area. (c) The San Francisco AIDS Foundation 1986, 1987.

it presents issues unlike others with which managers have had experience.

AIDS as a Disease

Much of our discussion about AIDS has focused on the macro picture, the epidemic, where AIDS came from, what path it has taken through the population, who it has affected to this point, and how it is transmitted. Understanding AIDS also requires comprehending the micro view, how the disease affects individual people, because not everyone with AIDS responds to the infection in exactly the same way.

AIDS, as defined by the Centers for Disease Control, is an immune-suppressed condition which (a) is not an inherited immune disorder like that of the so-called "Bubble Boy" in Houston a few years ago; (b) is not due to any immunosuppressive medical treatment such as the anti-rejection drugs given to organ transplant recipients; and (c), because of this immune deficiency, is characterized by infections with certain "opportunistic" diseases, those that are known to take advantage of the opportunity presented by the damaged immune system. A specific list of these opportunistic diseases has been drawn up by CDC, and it is this *list* that determines a diagnosis of AIDS. AIDS is not a disease in itself, but a condition in which the immune system is severely damaged by an invading virus; and, because of the damage to the immune system, the body is subject to infection and attack by *other* diseases.

As is the case with other diseases, infection with the AIDS virus can result in the full spectrum of illness, ranging from no symptoms at all to death from a variety of severe opportunistic infections. In the middle of this spectrum are mild to severe illnesses consisting of various nonspecific symptoms, including fever, fatigue, weight loss, diarrhea, and swollen lymph glands. These lesser symptoms are loosely categorized as AIDS-related Complex, or "ARC," medical conditions caused by the AIDS virus, but which do not match the CDC's specific requirements for an official diagnosis of AIDS.★

The difference between AIDS and ARC is largely a matter of definition and not necessarily a matter of severity of symptoms. The CDC has chosen to count only those people affected with specific opportunistic disease as having an AIDS diagnosis. For statistical purposes, only those people who fit the CDC definition of AIDS are included in the count of AIDS patients. The CDC does not track the number of people with ARC, although officials at the center are trying to find ways to accurately define and identify ARC cases. Estimates based on clinical observation indicate that there may be as many as ten cases of ARC for each diagnosed case of AIDS.

Some people whose bodies have been infected with the AIDS virus will display no symptoms at all for a number of years. Whether they can remain asymptomatic for the rest of their lives remains to be seen, although some physicians think it may be possible. Some of these infected people will develop symptoms and be diagnosed as having "ARC." They may remain in this condition for several years. Some people with ARC will require extensive medical treatment; others will not. Some ARC patients will be severely debilitated and disabled; others will be functional and able to carry on a normal life. Others with ARC will eventually progress to the stage meeting the CDC definition of AIDS. Still others will go from being asymptomatic to having full-blown AIDS.

The specific path that the disease may follow within an individual infected with the AIDS virus will vary substantially from person to person. The body's first response to the presence of the virus is the production of "antibodies." This usually occurs within a few weeks, or months, after infection. The infected person will

---

★*Acquired Immune Deficiency Syndrome in California: A Prescription for Meeting the Needs of 1990.* California Department of Health Services, Sacramento, March 1986.

be unaware of the production of these antibodies, which can be detected only in a blood test. The antibody test can serve as an early warning of viral infection, and can advise a person of his or her ability to transmit the virus to someone else through unprotected sexual intercourse or the sharing of needles. The antibody test has proven invaluable as a means of protecting the blood supply. It has also been useful in research settings to refine our understanding of how AIDS is and is not transmitted. Unlike antibodies produced against other diseases, antibodies to the AIDS virus seem to have no protective effect. Once an individual's immune system has been damaged by the virus to the point where an opportunistic disease can and does take hold, the condition is assumed to be fatal, with an average life expectancy of eighteen months.

Many of the specific opportunistic diseases experienced by AIDS patients can be successfully treated for a time. AIDS patients can often enjoy periods of good health. But the underlying loss of an effective immune system, and worse, the daily deterioration of the person's already weakened immune system, means that the opportunistic diseases will eventually return. On the positive side, a handful of people have managed to lead useful and relatively healthy lives for five or more years following diagnosis. More typically, persons diagnosed with AIDS will experience periods of good health, followed by a return of opportunistic infections, followed by more functional periods.

The employability of people with AIDS or ARC varies a great deal from individual to individual. AIDS patients are not a threat to anyone at work, so employers should offer them the same employment opportunities that would be available to employees with other illnesses. The degree to which a person might wish to work after such a diagnosis varies from employee to employee. For some people, work is extraordinarily important, and the continuation of work is an essential part of maintaining their health and of maximizing their life expectancy in the face of an ultimately fatal disease. For most employees with AIDS, continued work is almost always a financial necessity. The principle of "reasonable accommodation," of the kind organizations have applied to issues connected with the people who are disabled or handicapped would also apply, as a practical and·a legal matter, to people with AIDS and ARC.

3 ‖ Managing the Fear of Managing AIDS in the Workplace

For several decades now, employers have routinely managed issues of health and illness in the workplace. Whether in relation to employee safety, employee benefits, insurance costs, employee relations or compliance with a variety of laws, health is a regularly accepted topic of management interest. Sound employee health is often a recognized organizational goal. Many companies have comprehensive health care programs, extensive safety training programs and educational programs covering numerous specific occupational health risks at work. More employers now have well-financed and well-organized health promotion programs within the workplace, where employee interest in the topic of health is reasonably high. Nevertheless, the majority of business organizations, including many that are vulnerable to the issue of AIDS in the workplace, have not yet developed a planned organizational approach to *this* health topic.

In most organizations, there also exists a fairly complete context for dealing with a multitude of legal issues surrounding rights and obligations of employment, including issues of discrimination, equal employment opportunity and the physically handicapped. Organizations make a heavy investment in legal advice and routinely educate their management staffs about corporate legal obligations so that managers will avoid expensive and troublesome violations of law. As a general rule, though, most American business organizations have not yet prepared their staffs to deal specifically with the legal issues attached to AIDS.

In the most typical of such organizations, either AIDS is not yet seen as an appropriate area for corporate response, or other issues and attitudes, biases or fears, have interfered with the development of a response to AIDS. For many managers, the entire topic of AIDS is still filed away in a mental drawer labeled "this does not involve our workplace." In the face of evidence to the contrary and despite growing recognition of the harm AIDS can cause within a business organization when management is unprepared for it, too many organizations have done nothing whatever about AIDS. If your organization has avoided making a plan for AIDS, we suggest that you consider the typical barriers managers face when deciding on an AIDS policy. In reviewing the reasons most frequently cited by managers for not dealing with AIDS in the workplace, you will see that most excuses are usually rationalizations for unexpressed fears of various kinds.

Common Fears Associated with Managing AIDS in the Workplace

In our experience, there are four steps towards formulating an effective policy for dealing with AIDS in the real world of the workplace: (1) Recognize that AIDS is here and is a legitimate workplace issue; (2) learn what AIDS is; (3) understand why AIDS seems awkward and complicated, and admit why we fear it and want to avoid it; and (4) learn how to effectively manage it.

In October 1986, the United States Surgeon General, Dr. C. Everett Koop, issued the "Surgeon General's Report on Acquired Immune Deficiency Syndrome." In it, he recommended that ". . . work sites should have a plan in operation for education of the work force and accommodation of AIDS or ARC patients *before* the first such case appears at the work site." This official recognition of the relationship of AIDS to the American workplace by the nation's chief physician and his clear call for advance preparation by employers has produced for many organizations a major attitudinal shift towards AIDS.

Following the Surgeon General's recommendations and with the growing coverage of the AIDS issue in the business literature and on the programs of management seminars, managers in most industries, government agencies, and nonprofit organizations now recognize that the issue of AIDS cannot be avoided indefinitely, and that the cost of waiting for the issue to arise unexpectedly will inevitably exceed the cost of preparing for it. Yet there is remarkable resistance and procrastination among managers about the issue. In talking with managers who demonstrate varying degrees of "denial" about AIDS, we have observed that acknowledging the procrastination and admitting the reasons for it go a long way towards resolving the resistance and allowing for action on the issue. With this topic, facing our fears and telling the truth about them are essential first steps in solving the problem. Management *fears* about a number of issues associated with AIDS are the biggest stumbling block about which the truth needs to be told. Let's look at some of the most common fears that get in the way of preparing for AIDS.

Fear: What Has This Disease to Do with Us?

It is natural for human beings to avoid responding to any new stimulus unless it somehow affects them personally. For many people, AIDS is someone else's disease. They experience the AIDS epidemic as something remote, as something that affects other people, people who are "not like them." They see AIDS as something that affects only certain geographic regions of the country, as something that could not possibly take place within "their" environment. For people with highly depersonalized perspectives on this epidemic, AIDS is not seen as a widespread and growing international problem having the potential to attack any organization of any size in any location.

For managers resisting dealing with AIDS because of narrow or depersonalized perspectives on the disease, the solution is to seek additional information and take a broader look at the status of the disease in our culture.

Fear: AIDS Requires That We Discuss Taboo Subjects at Work

For managers who view sex, homosexuality and drugs as taboo subjects, it is easy to want to avoid dealing with AIDS. Employees may support this avoidance, afterall they are also uncomfortable about the topic. As an official workplace issue, sex is an awkward subject. Many managers and employees may joke about sex in the workplace; it is a human trait to joke about subjects that make us uncomfortable. Or we may talk about sex under only some conditions, or only with certain kinds of groups. Most people view sex as a private matter, a subject that is inappropriate for free public discussion, and one that does not fall under management's jurisdiction.

Our attitudes about sex often reflect our personal, religious or moral values. Those values tend to define or influence how we deal with sex and how we respond to the way other people deal with sex. Examples of our cultural difficulties with sex abound. Our society always has enormous problems, for example, agreeing on how to approach sex education for our children, either at home or in the schools. The topic of sex education itself generates highly emotional debate on both sides of the issue; consensus is virtually impossible to find. The subject of pornography invariably brings about heated arguments on both sides. People who are ordinarily quite logical and rational on most subjects can become lost in the emotions of the issues surrounding sex. Most of us find honest *private* discussions about sex to be *awkward*; we may find honest *public* discussions about sex to be *unthinkable*.

The AIDS epidemic has churned up new evidence of deep-seated and generally unexpressed fears about sex within our culture. Just beneath the surface in our society there is an unarticulated fear that if we speak openly and honestly about sex, especially in public and especially around children and adolescents, that open conversation will lead to promiscuity, adultery and homosexuality, which in turn will lead to the destruction of the nuclear family on which our society is based, which will lead to the destruction of our society and civilization as we know it. As with sex education, pornography, abortion and other sexual issues, our society is deeply divided on the dangers of public discussions about sex. Many people find this fear absurd, contrary to the evidence, and clearly unjustifiable, while others believe it to be quite real.

Another complication we experience in openly discussing sexual matters is that even our language tends to fail us when it comes to the topic of sex. The words we have to describe sexual interactions are either extremely clinical—medical terms drawn from the *Latin*—or "dirty" slang words that cannot be used in polite conversation or in the text of this book. The language provides us with too few words which convey the beauty, deep emotional connection, sensitivity and lovingness that can be elements of human sexual interaction.

Our tradition is that sexual discussions are off-limits in the workplace, except for whispered rumors and sly jokes. Sex recently appeared as an official workplace topic only in the legally-focused contexts of discrimination or of sexual harassment. Even in those contexts, the cultural reluctance to discuss the subject has complicated the resolution of the legal and social problems involved. It's hard to deal intelligently with something we can't even discuss.

In order for managers to discuss the disease of AIDS and its consequences in the workplace, there must be a willingness to speak to some degree about sex. It is difficult to explain a sexually transmitted disease without mentioning sex. As a person with a key role in that process within your organization, you may have to face your personal awkwardness about sex and your personal uncertainty about how to best deal with the topic on the job.

If dealing with sex isn't tough enough, AIDS inevitably brings up the topic of homosexuality. Public discussion of homosexuality, known until recently as "the love that dare not speak its name," is extraordinarily awkward for most people. It is worth noting that homosexuality is peripheral in a discussion of the topic of AIDS, since the purpose of the discussion is to educate employees about the viral disease and its implications for the workplace, not to educate them about homosexuality. Nevertheless, homosexuality is an especially difficult and embarrassing topic for heterosexual males, given the strong negative conditioning about homosexuality to which males are exposed in our culture. Female managers generally have less difficulty and embarrassment with this topic than do their male counterparts. Because they are not personally threatened by the issue, women managers often have greater success than do their male colleagues in developing and implementing AIDS policies in the workplace.

Fear: Employees Are Very Conservative and Have Traditional Values

The past two generations have witnessed significant cultural changes in the lives and sexual patterns of Americans. These changes influence not only the future course of AIDS, but also affect the receptivity of our workplace audience in learning about AIDS. America is no longer a nation of people exclusively engaged in long-term, monogamous heterosexual relationships. The demographics of our population have changed dramatically over the past half-century, and particularly so over the last decade.

Our society's image of the American family is now out-of-date by several generations. Amazingly, the prevailing image of the typical American family is of an adult male and an adult female, legally and faithfully married to one another, living together in a household that also contains one or more minor children produced by that marriage. The finest example of that image is the Cleaver family of 1950s television fame.

To the contrary, the statistically "typical" American family today is more likely to consist of a single parent, separated or divorced, raising children alone, trying to cope with dating, making a living, raising children and planning a future, all outside the context of the "traditional" monogamous relationship. Younger people now typically delay marriage until they are well into their twenties, and with the exception of a few conservative church leaders, no one seriously suggests that they avoid all sexual activity until marriage. With divorce rates in the U.S. near 50 percent of the rate of marriages, many people return to the "sexual marketplace" in the months preceding or following a divorce, even if they did not otherwise engage in premarital or extramarital affairs.

Whether one approves or disapproves of these cultural changes, it is a fact that millions of Americans frequently have sexual encounters outside of traditional monogamous relationships, and that millions of Americans engage in sexual activities with persons of the same gender, if only occasionally. Within marriages, it traditionally has been somewhat acceptable for the male partner to have outside sexual encounters; however, within recent years, the double-standard has become less tolerated. Because the variance between our traditional image and the realities of our lives can have deadly consequences, we need to design health and personnel policies and approaches to sexual and social issues within our organizations that truly reflect the realities of the ways our employees actually live.

Fear: Planning for AIDS Will Be Taken to Mean That an Employee Already Has AIDS

A fear frequently expressed by employers is that if they plan for AIDS or announce a policy about it, their employees will conclude that there has already been a diagnosis of AIDS in the workforce. That conclusion by employees, it is argued, will cause outrageous rumors, followed by disruption and panic among workers and perhaps even among customers. The resulting upset and confusion could cause employee walk-outs or the loss of business and create a seriously negative public image.

This fear is that employees automatically would be convinced that management's talking openly about the existence of AIDS or setting a policy about AIDS means that AIDS is already present in the workplace, and results in confusion, disruption, lost time, productivity and income. While it is possible that such a disastrous reaction might occur, as a practical matter, it just doesn't happen that way in real life. To the contrary, evidence from the experience of hundreds of organizations is that planned approaches minimize conflict and confusion. Employee panic resulting from a carefully planned and organized approach to AIDS is virtually unheard of.

What often underlies this kind of example is that these managers are themselves afraid of the subject of AIDS. They are concerned about their ability to handle the multitude of sensitive issues they see associated with AIDS. Their fear is evident by the strong assumptions they make about how people in the workplace will respond to information and policies about AIDS. These managers generally have not yet taken the steps necessary to learn about the disease, to learn about how AIDS impacts the workplace, to re-search the experience of other employers. They have not taken the time to allay their own worries and uncertainties. This is an example of how fearful management can unknowingly project its own fears onto employees, customers or the public, and in doing so, block any AIDS program that might otherwise be in the mak-ing. Their fear keeps the organization unprepared and vulnerable, and when AIDS finally comes along, their fears become a self-fulfil-ling prophecy.

It is clearly appropriate to be concerned about how employees will respond to the introduction of the subject of AIDS in the workplace. It would be extremely foolish to be insensitive as to how any issue might be viewed by the variety of stakeholders involved in any organization. All employees—and managers are also employees—are capable of having fears and concerns about AIDS during their first encounter with the disease itself, or to information about it, or to the task of making decisions about it. After all, this has been a central premise of this chapter. However, managers would do well to first address their own personal fears and discomfort. Only then can they effectively deal with their business concerns about AIDS, or with the legitimate concerns of the employees and other stakeholders.

The experiences of hundreds of organizations who, after careful planning and preparation, have faced AIDS in the workplace have been remarkably positive; examples are included throughout the remainder of the book. If there is a common surprise for the managers who face the AIDS issue honestly and directly, it is that a great many employees accept the issue so well, appreciate the information, and generally welcome the company having taken a clear and well-articulated stand about a controversial disease.

A tale of two telephone companies illustrates the point. Pacific Bell Telephone Company is the largest employer in California, a state that has more than 20 percent of the nation's AIDS cases. By extrapolation, Pacific Bell has more cases of AIDS among its workforce than any other company in the nation, and indeed Pacific Bell was hit by the disease in the earliest stages of the epidemic.

Pacific Bell developed a corporate response to AIDS early in the epidemic in which employees with AIDS receive the same benefits and treatment as employees with any other kind of disease, including reasonable accommodation if they wish to continue working. To implement that policy of treating AIDS like any other illness, Pacific Bell undertook an aggressive employee education program. The company newsletter frequently carried information about AIDS; educational forums featuring medical speakers were held for employees in locations all over the state; an excellent twenty-three-minute award-winning educational video about AIDS was produced by the corporate television department and was made available throughout the company. Trained counselors spoke with members of departments in which a co-worker was diagnosed. Pamphlets from various sources were widely distributed, and a company hotline was established to answer specific employee questions and concerns about AIDS.

The company backed its approach to AIDS with a well-organized, comprehensive employee education program in which both the disease and the company's response to the disease were explained in detail. Having determined its legal obligations based on the facts of this specific disease, the company actively sought employee cooperation. The result is that Pacific Bell has had a consistently superb record with its employees over this issue for several years. Problems associated with employees continuing to work after a diagnosis of AIDS have been few.

On the other hand, New England Bell Telephone had perhaps the most publicly disastrous experience with AIDS of any company in the country. When the company decided a couple of years ago that it had to allow a person diagnosed with AIDS to return to work, it treated the matter as a legal one. Because so many lawyers were dealing with the policy decisions, New England Telephone did not tie that policy decision into an organized employee communication and education program. As a result of the absence of coordinated and supportive education of co-workers, some New England Telephone employees refused to work even in the same facility with the AIDS patient; they walked off the job while the television cameras caught the entire story for the evening news.

The New England Telephone employee with AIDS was eventually returned to work, but not without a great deal of avoidable chaos, confusion and hard feelings between management and labor, in addition to expensive litigation, and a lot of embarrassing publicity for the company. New England Telephone used this problem to spearhead a progressive AIDS program and now is a leader in the Northeast in managing AIDS in the workplace.

The most striking instances of employee panic and negative publicity during the course of the AIDS epidemic have come from organizations that did not bother to learn about AIDS prior to its appearance in the workplace, those that did not take the opportunity to prepare in advance and those that did not consider the issues of human psychology necessary for a rational resolution of the matter. The reactive approach is virtually always ultimately more costly than the preventive approach.

Fear: Taking a Stand on AIDS Puts Us Uncomfortably on Record about a Moral Issue

Some people view AIDS as the result of "immoral behavior" and argue that society has no responsibility towards those who are reaping the consequences of such behavior. Some might even suggest that management has a specific moral obligation *not* to treat AIDS with compassion, because to do so would represent a corporate stamp of approval on "immoral conduct." Many managers express concern that investors or stockholders may not appreciate a policy that runs counter to their personal values.

To the contrary, a policy about AIDS need not be a stand about a moral issue at all. An AIDS policy focuses on a disease and its consequences in the workplace. To hold that the "moral" questions about AIDS obviates or alters any corporate, social or legal responsibility about this disease would be inconsistent with the legal system. In fact, it would be a remarkable violation of American business tradition. In the American business culture, and in your own corporate culture, management typically does not make "moral" judgments about *any* other health issue in the workplace. Injecting morality into the field of employee benefits and health policy would be a risky decision, especially when there inevitably will be a conflict between one person's view of the moral issue and the more objectively determinable responsibilities of the company under the applicable law.

Fear: If We Base a Policy on Existing Medical Information and the Information Turns Out to Be Wrong, We Could Be Liable

Updated medical and scientific information about AIDS is consistently reported and supported by the United States Public Health Service, the Surgeon General of the U.S., the Centers for Disease Control, the American Medical Association, the National Academy of Sciences and the World Health Organization. There is widespread agreement among researchers and academics from schools of medicine about how AIDS is spread. Employment policies based on that kind of scientific unanimity can be implemented with confidence. It is legally safe to act upon what is currently recognized as the body of scientific knowledge and upon the advice of the government agencies and officials who are charged with responsibility for disseminating the facts about this disease.

Fear: Our Employees Will Be Offended If We Bring Up the Subject of AIDS in the Workplace

As we have noted previously, managers planning an AIDS program need to examine their own feelings, concerns, beliefs and attitudes about AIDS to be certain they are not projecting their own issues onto their employees. In cases of serious doubt, there are a variety of techniques for assessing employees' reactions. Run a pilot project, conduct some surveys or select some employees for a focus group discussion. You will likely discover more openness than you anticipated, especially if your program is honest, well-conceived, mature and faces all the issues without embarrassment. Another way to assess whether or not employees want information on AIDS is to look at the experience of employers who have developed policies and provided information about

AIDS and see how their employees responded. It is our experience that employees recognize and appreciate the fact that it takes guts to face this issue forthrightly in the workplace.

Fear: AIDS Is Not a Workplace Issue; People's Private Lives Are None of Our Business

"You don't get AIDS at work, so why should we deal with AIDS at work?" This astonishing question was asked by a corporate medical department nurse who should know better. The principal focus of any program about AIDS in the workplace should be the workplace. Drawing the line between legitimate business concerns and the private lives of employees may be a difficult task, but it isn't an unreasonable intrusion into an employee's private life for an organization to develop policies and plans about the way a new epidemic could impact the workplace or about what a diagnosis of AIDS would mean on the job. Nor is it an intrusion to make available information on how employees can avoid exposure to AIDS off the job.

Even among companies which do not prohibit smoking on the job, few would suggest that providing information about the cancer risk of smoking is an intrusion into employees' private lives. Employees need to know about AIDS so that they can respond intelligently if a co-worker contracts the disease. Also, information about AIDS' risks should be passed along by employees to their insured dependents. The teenagers of America are generally covered for medical expenses under their parents' health insurance at work. Employers have a legitimate financial interest in AIDS' prevention for employees and their insured dependents.

Fear: We Don't Know How to Manage Our Employees' Fear of AIDS

Management routinely deals with employees' fears in the workplace. Employees can become frightened by any significant change in the work environment, from a new organizational structure, a new boss or a new assignment to a new computer system or major changes in work responsibility. Management often responds to employee fears with sympathy and patience, expressing a willingness to listen and to explain. Management often attempts to alleviate employee fears through educational programs, some of which may be quite elaborate, depending on the issues and the number of people affected. Most managers know how to recognize and deal with employee fear through education and communication. Good managers know that fear cannot be allowed to dictate organizational policy.

Fear: An AIDS Program Will Be Costly

In an era of tight cost control within American business, management may believe that the cost of an AIDS education program cannot be justified. Preparing and implementing AIDS programs within the organization need not cost a lot of money.

The cost of a comprehensive AIDS program can vary from a few hundred dollars to thousands of dollars, depending on the complexity of the program and the size and geographic distribution of the workforce. In situations where cost is a significant factor, it is still possible to implement an effective AIDS program. Many large companies already have effective AIDS programs in place and are generous about sharing information. There are now AIDS-related organizations in many communities that will assist employers in developing AIDS education programs. To help control costs, AIDS education can be tied in with existing health education or workplace safety programs.

Fear: Top Management Won't Like the Suggestion That We Plan for AIDS. This Issue Could Be Hazardous to My Career

Usually the impetus to develop an AIDS policy comes from people in middle management who are responsible for the day-to-day operation of the workplace. They are the front-line people who have to implement decisions in ways that comply with the law and protect the organization from costly litigation and employee relations problems. Personnel specialists, including human resource managers, employee assistance people, benefits managers, legal advisors, trainers, and safety experts have been among the first to recognize an organization's need to plan for AIDS.

AIDS is still controversial, and it is important that middle managers and human relations specialists get support from top management before proceeding with the development of a program. To get that support, they must communicate up through the various levels the reasons for dealing with AIDS. The people at the top have the power to advance or block careers. Some managers are reluctant to take on the AIDS issue because they are afraid it might damage their reputations or their careers. They worry that they will become *personally* suspect if they promote or encourage a corporate approach to the AIDS issue. They fear that they will be seen as sympathetic to homosexuals or drug users, or worse still, that they may be suspected of being homosexual. For managers who experience those fears, it is certainly tempting to avoid and ignore the entire topic.

In our experience, avoiding a management decision because of concerns about what others may think carries its own long-term career risks. The managers who have addressed the AIDS issue have occasionally encountered some resistance; however, those managers who persevered have usually succeeded in achieving their goals. They had to do their homework. They found it necessary to research what other organizations have done successfully or unsuccessfully. They identified the pitfalls and defined their goals, and selected effective strategies from the array available to them.

Most importantly, they effectively educated senior management about AIDS, about how the organization would benefit from an effective AIDS program, and about the risks of unpreparedness.

In the process, many of these managers found their perseverance and courage ultimately rewarded. We know of several managers who were promoted because of their courageous performance on the AIDS issue within their organizations. More than one executive have found leadership on the AIDS issue a path to career advancement.

4 || Step-by-Step Management of AIDS in the Workplace

The specific steps to developing an AIDS policy will vary from organization to organization. Size of the company, type of industry, geographic distribution and demographics of the workforce and corporate style will all help to determine how your organization deals with this issue. We recommend that you apply three general principles to everything you do regarding AIDS:

1. Manage AIDS the way you would manage any other workplace issue.
2. Do what you already know how to do.
3. Be consistent with your own organizational culture.

These principles are so obvious that many organizations overlook them. Mistakes made around management of the AIDS issue almost invariably involve a violation of one or more of these simple ideas.

It is seldom wise to try experimental approaches in setting policies about AIDS. If you are unhappy with the way your organization sets strategies and communicates with employees, or if you have been looking for a major issue to approach in a completely different way, please do not choose AIDS. Find a less controversial topic with which to experiment.

There is nothing innately unique about AIDS that calls for a different approach. AIDS, like any other new problem in the environment, requires that you learn about it and evaluate how it might impact your business. You gather together the appropriate people and plan a response based on the facts, the law and the economic and human factors.

AIDS is fundamentally no different from any other new issue. Treating it as something extraordinary invariably leads to difficulty. Manage AIDS the way you would any other issue on the job. Stick with familiar processes and tested methodologies that employees have learned to expect. Do what you already know works in your organization, and act consistently within your organizational style and culture.

While it is always preferable that you handle AIDS within the familiar processes of your organization, it is also important that whatever you do regarding AIDS be done extremely well. This is not an issue to be treated sloppily or with casual indifference.

The challenge of managing AIDS presents a superb opportunity for your organization to demonstrate how well it can work. A sense of pride in having tackled a tricky new management issue, and having done so with wisdom, courage and intelligence, will be communicated throughout your organization and will establish a receptive environment for the approach to AIDS you have selected.

Getting Started

Someone within the organization must take responsibility for initiating a response to AIDS. With the assistance of one or more colleagues and with the approval of one or more higher-ups within the organization, someone must serve as the "Source" of an organizational approach to AIDS. The "Source" need not be the person with ultimate authority to set policy, but more likely will be the individual within the organization who has responsibility for seeing that the task is carried out. The specific job title of the Source and his or her position within the organizational structure will vary from one organization to another; however, the Source must exist or nothing will happen.

In some cases, a group might serve as the Source of a prepared approach to AIDS. More commonly, one individual will have been the Source of the group. Very often the person who provides the energy behind development of a corporate policy to AIDS is also the person most likely to be blamed should a crisis erupt over AIDS without the organization's having been prepared for it. There is nothing wrong with that method of selection; it is arguably the method by which most things get done in most organizations most of the time. If that is the way a "Source" is usually selected in your organization, then do what you normally do. Otherwise, recognize that someone has to take primary responsibility for this issue, and proceed accordingly.

Five Steps To a Planned Approach to AIDS

There are five key steps in developing a planned approach to AIDS in the workplace.

1. Define your organizational point of view about AIDS.

2. Determine whether a formal policy about AIDS is needed, and if so, what kind of policy is preferable.

3. Decide how, to whom and under what circumstances there will be communication about the organization's point of view about AIDS.

4. Decide how, to whom and under what circumstances there will be education about AIDS—who within the organization will be educated about the disease, at what stages, and how that education will be achieved: (a) now, as part of the planning process; (b) later, as part of implementing the resulting plan;

(c) when a case of AIDS is diagnosed in the workforce; (d) as a matter of AIDS-prevention for anyone who might be sexually active or who might use IV drugs (that is, *all* employees).

5. Decide how the organization will respond to an AIDS crisis, now or in the future, and how the crisis will be resolved: (a) Who will be called upon; (b) what will be done; (c) what resources are available; and (d) how decisions will be made and carried out.

It may not be necessary for your organization to establish a formal policy about AIDS. We argue for planning a corporate response, for being prepared, for educating key people in advance and for knowing what you are going to do before you have to do it. On the other hand, not every organization needs a formal policy in order to be prepared.

An organization should know in advance what its approach to AIDS will be. Some minimum number of key people need to understand the medical facts about AIDS, know the organizational viewpoint about AIDS should it occur in your workplace, and be equipped to educate others about both the disease and your policy.

Establish a Task Force to Plan for AIDS

One of the best approaches to prepare for AIDS in the workplace is to establish a planning task force. Include on the task force committee all the key stakeholders necessary to successfully carry out the plan. Some candidates to include on a task force are representatives from such departments as human resources, legal, medical, employee assistance, benefits, equal employment, public relations, training, employee communications and labor relations. It is best to include representatives from all appropriate departments and unions as this is not an issue on which you want to invite sideline sabotage from elements of the organization who were left out of the process.

On the other hand, a huge task force representing everyone can be unworkable. Work with a group large enough to represent all the various essential interests yet small enough to still be manageable. Set a timetable by which the task force is to complete its work, and bear in mind that the task force's work must be managed.

Whether the members of the planning task force will be appointed from above or cooperatively assembled on a horizontal basis will depend on the organization's structure and style and on who is providing the leadership. To the extent possible, make certain that the representatives on the committee are individuals who have the courage of their convictions, and who have track records of influence within their own departments. The task force will need people who can sell the committee's decisions to other departments. The members' credibility and standing within the organization will be important. This task force should represent as good a team as your organization is capable of assembling, a selection of your best and most respected people.

Determine the Organization's
Point of View About AIDS

The first of the five steps required in a planned approach to AIDS is determining your organization's point of view about the disease. The task force should consider (a) the medical facts about the disease and how it is and is not transmitted; (b) the legal issues which will affect how much freedom you have in dealing with AIDS; (c) cost considerations; and (d) basic organizational philosophy about values, relationships with employees and civic responsibility.

The scientific and medical facts about AIDS are by now established. Tens of thousands of AIDS cases over many years uniformly fit into predictable patterns. AIDS is not spread by ordinary workplace interactions. The only alternative point of view would be based on the idea that "we don't yet know enough about this disease." Concern about contagion in the workplace could only come either from the most unusually conservative theories of medicine at the extreme ends of the spectrum, or from a perspective about transmission that, if correct, means AIDS is so easily spread that everyone is going to get it eventually, so there isn't much point to prevention or education.

Those who constantly raise issues of "what if" to justify keeping AIDS patients out of the workplace do so out of fear, ignorance or simple bias. The same "what if" point of view could be used with equal validity to justify keeping people with heart disease or breast cancer or Hodgkin's disease or sickle cell anemia out of the workforce. After all, no one has really *proven* you can't catch cancer from a co-worker. What if the evidence just hasn't turned up yet?

Some people may not like many of the people who have thus far contracted AIDS. Some people may not approve of the activities that spread AIDS. Liking or disliking people or activities cannot justify an organization's adopting a point of view about the disease that flies in the face of scientific reality.

Consider the Medical Facts   Chief among the many public health authorities who have spoken out about AIDS, the Surgeon General of the United States seems to have made the clearest statement:

> Everyday living does not present any risk of infection. You cannot get AIDS from casual social contact. Casual social contact should not be confused with casual sexual contact which is a major cause of the spread of the AIDS virus. Casual social contact such as shaking hands, hugging, social kissing, crying, coughing or sneezing, will not transmit the AIDS virus. Nor has AIDS been contracted from swimming in pools or bathing in hot tubs or from eating in restaurants (even if a restaurant worker has AIDS or carries the AIDS virus). AIDS is not contracted from sharing bed linens, towels, cups, straws, dishes, or any other eating utensils. You cannot get AIDS from toilets, doorknobs, telephones, office machin-

ery, or household furniture. You cannot get AIDS from body massages, masturbation or any non-sexual contact.

No medical or scientific researcher of AIDS has ever expressed, based on any claim of scientific evidence or logic, another point of view about transmission of this disease. The only argument to the contrary is based exclusively on "what ifs," not one of which has occurred in all these years. Rational people do not make decisions about their lives or their businesses based on avoiding "what if" situations that have never occurred, and that have no scientific support for a prediction of occurrence.

There is no medical or scientific basis for excluding a person with AIDS from the workplace. The evidence overwhelmingly supports the view that AIDS is not a threat in the workplace for employees as long as they engage in the activities they are paid to perform. If irrational fears were present about any other new issue on the job, education and counseling would be used to manage those fears. AIDS should be managed the same way other issues are managed.

Consider the Legal Issues Legal advice tends to become quickly outdated with the passage of new legislation, and as each new court decision or administrative ruling is handed down. Many organizations arguably receive far too much legal advice already. Nevertheless, there are important legal issues that form part of the overall picture of AIDS in the workplace. Obtaining good current legal advice is an important part of determining a point of view about the disease.

Legal counsel will probably advise you that, under federal and state laws, AIDS should be treated as a legal handicap or disability against which you cannot legally discriminate and for which you are obligated to provide reasonable accommodation. Counsel also will probably suggest that if you operate in one of several cities or states in which specific AIDS antidiscrimination legislation has been passed, you risk fines or criminal penalties for employment practices that discriminate against persons with this disease. In all likelihood, you will be advised that you have an obligation to treat employees equally, in the absence of some reasonable basis for treating them differently. If you have certain benefits available to people with leukemia or Parkinson's disease, you had best be prepared to demonstrate why you should treat employees with AIDS differently.

You can expect to be advised that medical information provided in confidence by an employee to the employer is confidential. The employer has no right, and in the case of AIDS no responsibility, to disclose that information to other workers. Good legal counsel may also advise you that while the AIDS virus isn't hazardous to your corporate health, discrimination litigation may be.

Union contracts often specifically protect workers who are physically able to work. Labor unions have provided leadership in the protection of AIDS patients in America, Canada, England and Australia. Unions are often excellent sources of educational materials and information about AIDS. People with AIDS have won most of the cases actually litigated over AIDS discrimination, even though many did not live to witness their legal victory. Unions have often provided the continuity behind such litigation when the employee is unable to do so. Trends in labor law are moving towards protection of the ill employee. Recently, the U.S. Supreme Court ruled that a person with tuberculosis—a conventionally contagious disease, whereas AIDS is not conventionally contagious—is legally protected in the workplace.

Set Forth the Facts   An organizational point of view about AIDS might include the following statements:

- AIDS is a relatively new disease caused by a virus that is infecting millions of people worldwide.

- Tens of thousands of Americans are already diagnosed with

AIDS, and U.S. Public Health officials estimate that at least one quarter of a million more Americans will be diagnosed with AIDS by the early 1990s.

- The overwhelming scientific evidence as stated by the U.S. Public Health Service, the Centers for Disease Control, the Surgeon General of the United States and other health experts consulted by this company is that AIDS is spread by sexual intercourse with an infected person or by direct contact between the bloodstream of an infected person and the bloodstream of another, or by maternal transmission from an infected woman to her unborn child.

- AIDS is not a risk in our workplace while employees are engaged in work activity; therefore, there is no reason why a person diagnosed with AIDS cannot continue to work as long as he or she is physically able to meet acceptable job performance standards. The clear trend among employers is to treat AIDS like any other life-threatening illness such as cancer or heart disease.

- Legal requirements tend to uphold the right of a person with AIDS to be employed if he or she is able to perform the work. AIDS appears to be a legally protected handicap/disability under state and federal laws.

- The experience of other companies indicates that uninformed co-workers can become frightened if a colleague on the job is diagnosed with AIDS. This fear complicates what would otherwise be a fairly straightforward matter; therefore, employers are finding it necessary to implement education programs about the disease.

- The Surgeon General of the United States recommends that employers have a plan in place about AIDS *before* the first case of AIDS appears in the workforce.

Such statements form the basis for a point of view about AIDS, and present the organization's rationale for taking some action in the future. These factual statements also form the basis for future communications about whatever action you choose to take. The stated point of view need not declare what you're going to do about AIDS, although it may reveal the general direction of future actions. The importance of the point-of-view statement is that it lays out the *context* for decisions and action. It forms the framework for educating others about the disease, or about whatever action you subsequently decide to take.

Brief Top Management   At some point it will be useful to brief top management about the task force's work. The support of top management will be necessary if you are to successfully carry out *any* approach to the AIDS epidemic. Exactly how the briefing should be handled and who needs to be included will depend on the individual organization. In some companies, Bank of America, for example, the Board of Directors was briefed on the epidemic and the company's response to it. In other organizations, the chief human resources official serves as top management for the briefing. Typically, though, the CEO is the top official to be included in the process, unless there is also a board or management committee charged with jurisdiction over human resources issues. Your task force should determine how best to include top management in the process.

The briefing of top management might await completion of the task force's review of all aspects of AIDS and of detailed proposals for an overall corporate response. Another, and often preferred, option is to phase in the briefing process to give management an opportunity to absorb the facts and implications about AIDS in an orderly process over time. For example, once the task force has completed the development of a corporate point of view about AIDS, based on a review of the facts and the law, it might then be useful to give top management a briefing about just those matters. It's a way of saying "the AIDS epidemic is happening; here's what it looks like; we are working out what we should do about it; you'll be hearing more from us."

Review Existing Policies and Consider Options

A first step in considering what kind of policy, if any, you should have about AIDS is to examine what kinds of policies you already have in place. Make an inventory of existing policies covering issues like eligibility for medical benefits, long-term disability benefits, handicaps or physical disability on the job, reasonable accommodation and access to employee assistance programs. Your legal counsel will probably advise that you aren't required to have formal policies about many issues, but if you choose to have policies, you must apply them fairly and uniformly. Published policies are generally considered part of the contract between an organization and its workers. Make certain you have identified existing policies that might be applicable to AIDS before considering whether additional policies are necessary.

After educating yourself and reviewing the facts of AIDS and the legal environment in which you operate, and after determining your basic point of view about AIDS and taking an inventory of existing organizational policies, you next can consider whether you want to have an official policy about AIDS, and if so what kind of policy might be best for your situation. Most organizations tend to take one of four approaches to AIDS policies. The first approach is to do nothing about AIDS. Admittedly, some organizations may get away with doing nothing for several years, but the approach is an unnecessary gamble carrying potentially serious and expensive consequences should AIDS appear within that workforce.

The other approaches to AIDS policies tend to fall into one of three basic categories:

1. The "life-threatening illness" approach;
2. the "AIDS-specific" approach; or
3. the "deliberate no-policy" approach.

Variations on these three themes can be found in businesses, government agencies and nonprofit organizations across the country. Some policies are a blend of two approaches. Some organizations consider their employment policies to be a private matter of contract between the company and its employees. As a matter of course, such organizations do not make public their internal personnel policies, and in that spirit would not make public their internal policies on AIDS. Out of respect for that position, the policies cited here are those that have been made public or for which we have express permission to disclose, or those for which the organization's name has been deleted.

The Life-Threatening Illness Policy Approach Bank of America, one of the world's largest banks, first officially faced AIDS in 1983. A male employee in its California headquarters was hospitalized for a few weeks. When his physical condition improved, he advised his supervisor that (a) he and his doctor agreed he was ready to return to work; and (b) he had AIDS. With the best of intentions, but without considering the blatant disregard of the employee's confidentiality, the supervisor called in his co-workers and explained that John (not his real name) had AIDS and was coming back to work. The supervisor asked for their support of John through his difficult experience.

A few of the departmental employees were not in a mood to be supportive of John's return to work. At that time, AIDS was still a relatively new disease, and there was little certainty about its cause or means of transmission. As luck would have it, two of the female employees in the department were pregnant. They were especially concerned about John's presence in their work area. The father of one of the pregnant women was a labor lawyer. In short order the Bank received formal notice it would be charged with not maintaining a safe working environment as required by OSHA, should John be a part of that working environment.

To cool things off while deciding what to do, the Bank persuaded the disgruntled employees to take a paid leave for a few days. The Human Resources people then contacted the Centers for Disease Control in Atlanta, and consulted with local Health Department, hospital and occupational medical specialists. The Human Resources people heard the same opinion from each agency they consulted: although the disease was relatively new, the evidence was clear that AIDS was a sexually transmitted and blood-borne disease that would not be spread by ordinary workplace interactions. Fears to the contrary were understandable, but could not be justified under the known scientific facts about the disease. Co-workers were not at risk for AIDS.

The Bank concluded that they could find no medical justification for treating AIDS differently than they would any other disease, that having an employee with AIDS on the job was not a threat to co-workers, and that allowing an employee with AIDS in the workplace would not support a charge of failing to maintain a safe place for co-workers to work.

The dissident employees were advised that they were to return to work, and most of them did so. The OSHA claim was not pursued and no litigation resulted. The employee with AIDS returned to his office and continued to work without further incident until his health again deteriorated.

This experience led the Bank of America to consider what approach it should take towards AIDS in the likelihood that other of its more than 50,000 employees would be diagnosed with the disease. The point of view developed, and later approved at Board level, was that since there was no medical reason to treat AIDS differently from other major illnesses, an AIDS-specific policy was neither necessary nor appropriate. Instead, the Bank chose to reaffirm its approach to life-threatening illness in general. A policy statement about life-threatening illness, citing AIDS, cancer and heart disease as specific examples, was prepared by their task force.

The resulting statement (from *Assisting Employees with Life Threatening Illnesses*, Bank of America, revised October 1985) is an excellent example of a life-threatening illness approach to AIDS:

> BankAmerica recognizes that employees with life-threatening illnesses including but not limited to cancer, heart disease and AIDS may wish to engage in as many of their normal pursuits as their condition allows, including work. As long as these employees are able to meet acceptable performance standards, and medical evidence indicates that their conditions are not a threat to themselves or to others, managers should be sensitive to their conditions and ensure that they are treated consistently with other employees. At the same time, BankAmerica has an obligation to provide a safe work environment for all employees and customers. Every precaution should be taken to ensure that an employee's condition does not present a health and/or safety threat to other employees or customers.
>
> Consistent with this concern for employees with life-threatening illnesses, BankAmerica offers the following range of resources available through Personnel Relations:
>
> - Management and employee education and information on terminal illness and specific life-threatening illnesses.
> - Referral to agencies and organizations which offer supportive services for life-threatening illnesses.
> - Benefit consultation to assist employees in effectively managing health, leave and other benefits.
>
> **Guidelines:** When dealing with situations involving employees with life-threatening illnesses, managers should:
>
> 1. Remember that an employee's health condition is personal and confidential, and reasonable precautions should be taken to protect information regarding an employee's health condition.
> 2. Contact Personnel Relations if you believe that you or other employees need information about terminal illness, or a specific life-

threatening illness, or if you need further guidance in managing a situation that involves an employee with a life-threatening illness.

3. Contact Personnel Relations if you have any concern about the possible contagious nature of an employee's illness.

4. Contact Personnel Relations to determine if a statement should be obtained from the employee's attending physician that continued presence at work will pose no threat to the employee, co-workers or customers. BankAmerica reserves the right to require an examination by a medical doctor appointed by the company.

5. If warranted, make reasonable accommodation for employees with life-threatening illnesses consistent with the business needs of the division/unit.

6. Make a reasonable attempt to transfer employees with life-threatening illnesses who request a transfer and are experiencing undue emotional stress.

7. Be sensitive and responsive to co-workers' concerns, and emphasize employee education available through Personnel Relations.

8. No special consideration should be given beyond normal transfer requests for employees who feel threatened by a co-worker's life-threatening illness.

9. Be sensitive to the fact that continued employment for an employee with a life-threatening illness may sometimes be therapeutically important in the remission or recovery process, or may help to prolong that employee's life.

10. Employees should be encouraged to seek assistance from established community support groups for medical treatment and counseling services. Information on these can be requested through Personnel Relations or Corporate Health.

Similar approaches can be found at Chevron Corporation, Citibank, IBM, AT&T, Wells Fargo Bank, Syntex Corporation, Westinghouse, TransAmerica Corporation, Motorola, Phillips-Van Heusen and many lesser-known organizations who have adopted, often verbatim, a policy statement issued by one of the larger companies. The focus of these policies is life-threatening illness in general. If AIDS is mentioned at all, it is usually cited simply as one example of the kinds of illness addressed by the policy. The advantage of this approach is that it is consistent with the notion that AIDS is simply another disease. It affirms the employer's interest in all major life-threatening illnesses without appearing to single out or discriminate in favor of any specific illness.

Many other examples of life-threatening illness policies can be found. Most of them explicitly refer to AIDS, despite their seemingly generic approach. For example, a major computer manufacturer issued a statement to managers entitled "Life Threatening Illness Guidelines." The statement began:

> Over the past several years, employers have been besieged with legal problems regarding actions they have taken that involve employees. One of the areas that has received considerable attention is treatment of employees with life-threatening illnesses such as cancer, AIDS, heart disease and the like. Although [the company] has not experienced problems around this subject, [the company] feels that it would be helpful to get some information out to managers proactively rather than finding ourselves in a position to have to react in the future.

The balance of the one-page policy statement covered such items as the confidentiality of information about any employee's health, the need for sensitivity "to the possibility that co-workers may have very emotional reactions and express fear about working with an employee with a life-threatening illness," and the importance of making decisions that "are good business decisions and good people decisions." Managers were invited to contact Human Resources for information about specific diseases, including their "possible contagious nature," or for guidance in managing a given situation. As to employees' fears, "make a reasonable attempt to accommodate co-workers' requests for transfer, but give them no special consideration that would not be given to an employee not in this situation. Any transfer should also be consistent with the business needs of [the company.]"

Drug manufacturer Syntex's approach was to issue a single-page life-threatening illness statement entitled "Illness in the Workplace, A Syntex Management Philosophy" covering "life-threatening and/or catastrophic diseases, such as AIDS, cancer, multiple sclerosis, etc. . . ." The statement notes that "the policies and practices outlined here apply to other such disabilities, and do not change any existing medical, benefits or employee relations policies covering sickness or other disabilities."

The final paragraph of the Syntex statement, after outlining what the company will do about reasonable accommodation, benefits, confidentiality and co-worker sensitivity for life-threatening illnesses, refers specifically to AIDS:

> Due to unique concerns raised by the AIDS issue, the company will implement an educational program based on the best currently available medical knowledge to help employees understand what AIDS is and what it is not; how it is transmitted; and what policies the company has in place to cover employees with all disabilities, including AIDS.

The medical department of Pittsburgh-based Westinghouse Electric has been issuing periodic information packages about AIDS to its management for several years. A statement to Westinghouse Medical and EAP personnel from Corporate Medical Director E. C. Curtis, M.D., M.P.H., in 1986 explained:

> We are frequently asked, "What is our policy regarding AIDS?" The guidance we provide is as follows: Just as we have no special policy for dealing with employees who develop TB or tetanus, or who experience life-threatening trauma, we see no need for a separate specific policy regarding those who contract AIDS.

After discussing issues of reasonable accommodation, confidentiality and the need for medical case management of AIDS cases, the two-page statement concludes: "Westinghouse views AIDS as an illness, not as a crime or a punishment. We encourage compassion for the victims, and the provision of accurate appropriate information to all employees as an antidote to ungrounded fears and unreasoning exaggerations."

The AIDS-Specific Policy Approach   Wells Fargo Bank, one of the first organizations to address the issue of AIDS in the workplace, concluded that:

> The purpose of the AIDS policy is to reassure employees that *AIDS is not spread through casual contact* during normal work practices and to reduce unrealistic fears about contracting an AIDS virus-related condition. This policy also protects the legal rights of employees to work who are diagnosed with an AIDS virus-related condition and provides guidelines to manage employees or situations where infection with the AIDS virus is suspected. Wells Fargo's policy encourages supervisors to convey sensitivity and understanding to employees affected with a condition of the AIDS virus.

Morrison & Foerster is a large, prestigious law firm with offices in San Francisco, Los Angeles, Denver and Washington, D.C. By 1987, despite being located in four unusually high-risk cities, the firm had not encountered a single case of AIDS among its staff of nearly 800 people. Nevertheless, after several years of advising its corporate clients about AIDS, the firm decided to develop an internal AIDS policy and launched an ambitious firmwide education program designed to inform every member of its professional and nonprofessional staff in four cities about AIDS. Management of the firm elected to focus their policy specifically on the AIDS epidemic.

> Morrison & Foerster recognizes that Acquired Immune Deficiency Syndrome (AIDS), its related conditions such as AIDS Related Complex (ARC), and persons with seropositive test results pose significant and delicate

issues for employees in the workplace. Accordingly, we have established the following guidelines for handling employee issues that arise when an employee is affected by this disease.

1. The firm is committed to maintaining a safe and healthy work environment for all employees.
2. Consistent with this commitment, the firm will treat AIDS the same as other illnesses in terms of all our employee policies and benefits, such as group health and life insurance, disability leaves of absence and other disability benefits.
3. Based on the overwhelming preponderance of available medical and scientific opinion, including statements from the U.S. Public Health Service and the Centers for Disease Control, there is no evidence that the AIDS virus is casually transmitted in ordinary social or occupational settings or conditions. Therefore, subject to changes in available medical information, it is the policy of the firm that employees with AIDS or any of its related conditions may continue to work and the firm will provide them with reasonable accommodation as long as they are medically able to perform the duties of their position. Employees who are affected by AIDS or any other life-threatening illness will be treated with compassion and understanding in dealing with their personal crisis. Co-workers will be expected to not refuse to work or withhold their services for fear of contracting AIDS by working with an AIDS-affected person, and to not harass or otherwise discriminate against an AIDS-affected employee.
4. Recognizing the need for all employees to be able to be accurately informed about AIDS, the firm will make every effort to have information available regarding the facts about this disease, how it is transmitted and not transmitted, and how best to contain it from spreading. Employees who would like to be provided with this information should contact the Personnel Department.
5. Employees affected by AIDS or any of its related conditions or concerned about AIDS are encouraged to contact their supervisor, the Personnel Manager, or their Office Manager to discuss their concerns

and to obtain additional information. [Next followed names, addresses and phone numbers of AIDS organizations in San Francisco, Los Angeles, Washington and Denver.]

6. The firm will treat all medical information obtained from employees with AIDS or any of its related conditions confidentially as required by law.

Morrison & Foerster reserves the right to change this policy or make appropriate revisions, additions, amendments or corrections. We will notify you of any substantive changes.

If you have any questions about this policy or its interpretation or the information upon which it is based, please contact your Supervisor, the Personnel Manager, or your Office Manager.

Similarly, an independent government agency involved in forest management developed this kind of AIDS-specific policy:

We recognize AIDS as a health issue in American society that requires responsible organizations, including employers, to take positive actions to support efforts to educate the American public about risks, prevention approaches, and the basic human and civil rights of individuals suffering from this disease. Employers have an obligation to ensure that members of their workforce recognize that this disease is not spread by casual contact in the work environment. Therefore, workers who are known AIDS carriers need not be restricted from working, nor do carriers of the AIDS virus need to refrain from sharing the following facilities or equipment with their co-workers [followed by a list of typical equipment used in that agency, including restrooms and drinking fountains].

The above guidelines are well supported by the medical and research community. Based on these guidelines [the agency] recognizes that employees with life-threatening illness such as AIDS may wish to engage in as many of their normal pursuits as their condition allows, including work. As long as an employee is able to meet acceptable standards, and medical evidence indicates that their condition is not a threat to others, we will be sensitive to their condition, make reasonable accommodations, and ensure that they are treated consistently with other employees with respect for their need for confidentiality and basic human rights.

Pacific Gas and Electric Company, like Bank of America, was another large employer forced to deal with AIDS during the earliest stages of the epidemic. After its experience with the disease, the public utility company issued an AIDS-specific policy statement and set of guidelines. The several-page policy statement indicated that "based on extensive research into the subject and consultation with health experts in the field, the Company's position is that employees afflicted with AIDS do not present a health risk to other employees in the workplace under normal working conditions." The policy statement acknowledges that "several PG&E employees have contracted or died of AIDS."

In general, the policy provides that "employees afflicted with AIDS should be treated the same as any other Company employee." If co-workers become concerned about working with someone who has been diagnosed with AIDS, supervisors are asked to explain that casual contact at work poses no threat of transmission. "If necessary, supervisors should contact an appropriate Employee Assistance Program counselor to arrange for more comprehensive educational efforts of the workforce." The policy statement concludes with a set of questions and answers about AIDS.

PG&E, like Wells Fargo Bank, Levi Strauss, Crowley Maritime Corporation and other organizations, relies heavily upon educational efforts and counseling by employee assistance departments where necessary to calm specific co-worker fears, in addition to providing counseling to the employee with AIDS.

The Deliberate No-Policy Approach   Oddly enough, some of the organizations which most aggressively pursue policies of nondiscrimination about AIDS, and who are most supportive of employees when they are diagnosed with AIDS, do not have AIDS policies as such. If you ask officials of Levi Strauss, for example, about its policy, you'll be told they don't have a policy about AIDS. If you ask a manager of Pacific Bell Telephone, a company with a track record of successfully handling a larger number of diagnosed cases of AIDS in their workforce than any other company in the world, to describe their policy about AIDS, you'll be told that they don't have a policy about AIDS one way or the other.

Neither Levi Strauss nor Pacific Bell is dodging the issue, but instead has taken the view that AIDS does not require a special policy, or even an elaboration of an old policy. Both companies have policies about illness; AIDS is an illness. Both companies have policies about benefits, disability, reasonable accommodation, discrimination and employee assistance. Both companies have impressive tract records in handling AIDS-related issues in the workplace. Perhaps it is because of their aggressive companywide educational programs about the disease, and the clarity of their points of view about AIDS, that this approach has been so workable.

The no-policy policy carries risks of confusion. Some companies say they have no policy about AIDS when what they really mean is that they don't know what their policy is. A no-policy policy seems to work only when the organization has a clear and well-articulated point of view that AIDS patients are entitled to work, that employees' fears of working with an infected person are groundless and that discrimination against AIDS patients won't be tolerated. Otherwise, there is the real possibility that "no-policy" means "no decision."

The Chamber of Commerce Model Approach   As a service to its members and as a model for employers, the San Francisco Chamber of Commerce in 1987 developed a recommended approach to AIDS in the workplace. Based on a review of local employers' extensive experience with the disease, and after considering approaches taken elsewhere in the country, the policy statement was developed by a task force headed by Dr. Julius Kevans, distinguished Chancellor of the University of California's state medical complex. The policy statement (from the San Francisco Chamber of Commerce, *AIDS in the Workplace: Suggested Guidelines for the Business Community*, June 1987) reads as follows:

> Epidemics of disease present enormous dilemmas to our society, straining our human, financial and health resources. Like smallpox, cancer and polio before it, Acquired Immune Deficiency Syndrome (AIDS) and its related conditions are approaching pandemic proportions. The impact of AIDS is and will continue to be devastating. According to the Surgeon General of the United States:

> *By the end of 1991, an estimated 270,000 cases of AIDS will have occurred with 179,000 deaths within the decade since the disease was first recognized. In the year 1991, an estimated 145,000 patients with AIDS will need health and supportive services at a total cost between $8 billion and $16 billion. However, AIDS is preventable. It is the responsibility of every citizen to be informed about AIDS and to exercise the appropriate prevention measures.*

> If we are to overcome the obstacles presented by AIDS and its related conditions, it is imperative that we respond immediately as a unified society. A comprehensive and effective approach toward combatting the epidemic only can be realized through a national effort with the full support, understanding and informed decision-making of the business community. Any sensible and humane response to the epidemic must be based on accurate information, not irrational fear and discrimination. There is an alarming tendency to label people as belonging to AIDS "risk groups." This is not only misleading, it is dangerous. AIDS is not confined to any single community. It is not caused by life-style or sexual orientation. It is caused by a virus—a virus that can be transmitted

to anyone who engages in high-risk activity. Fortunately, by modifying these high-risk behaviors, we can stop virus transmission. Unlike many other life-threatening illnesses, AIDS can be prevented.

We are fighting a disease, not people. The business community in America can and must play a major role in creating policies and disseminating accurate information about AIDS and its related conditions.

Any employee with a life-threatening and/or catastrophic illness such as AIDS, cancer or multiple sclerosis should be treated in conjunction with the principles outlined below. It is our desire that every business in America adopt and/or incorporate these principles into personnel policies and adhere to the content and spirit of the principles.

1. Employees with any life-threatening illness should be offered the right to continue working so long as they are able to continue to perform their job satisfactorily and so long as the best available medical evidence indicates that their continual employment does not present a health or safety threat to themselves or others.
2. Employers and co-workers should treat all medical information obtained from employees with strict confidentiality. In the case of an employee with a life-threatening illness, confidentiality of employee medical records in accordance with existing legal, medical, ethical and management practices should be maintained.
3. Employees who are affected by any life-threatening illness should be treated with compassion and understanding in their personal crisis. Reasonable efforts should be made to accommodate seriously ill patients by providing flexible work areas, hours and assignments whenever possible or appropriate.
4. Employees should be asked to be sensitive to the needs of critically ill colleagues, and to recognize that continual employment for an employee with a life-threatening illness is often life sustaining and can be both physically and mentally beneficial.
5. In regard to the life-threatening disease of AIDS and its related conditions, a person carrying the AIDS virus is not a threat to co-workers since AIDS is not spread by common everyday contact. For this reason,

the AIDS antibody and/or AIDS virus status of an employee is not relevant information in regard to the health and safety of his/her co-workers. Therefore, the AIDS antibody test and/or AIDS virus test should not be used as a prerequisite for employment or a condition for continued employment. Knowledge or presumed knowledge of AIDS antibody and/or AIDS virus status should not be used to discriminate against an employee for any reason.

6. Given the irrational fear that AIDS, cancer and other life-threatening diseases often inspire, the most effective way to avoid necessary disruptions in the workplace is to prepare and educate both management and employees before any employee is affected by a life-threatening disease. To this end, employers should implement educational programs based on the best available medical knowledge to understand the disease; what services are locally available to help employees with any medical, psychological or financial hardships caused by the disease, and what policies the company has in place to cover employees with a life-threatening illness.

Business and professional organizations have consistently helped to disseminate useful advice about AIDS to their memberships. "AIDS in the workplace" is a frequent workshop topic at meetings of such groups as the American Bankers Association, the American Society for Training and Development, the Equal Employment Advisory Council and industry groups like the Edison Electric Institute.

The formation in 1987 of the National Leadership Coalition on AIDS, composed of corporations, trade and professional associations, academic institutions, community-based nonprofit, and labor, minority, and religious groups, is intended to further "mobilize the resources of the private sector in the fight against AIDS," and actively promote additional joint efforts among business and labor organizations. Businesses seem instinctively to understand that so long as the media continues to stir up paranoia about AIDS, and so long as both the legal requirements and scientific facts support treating AIDS like any other disease, intercompany cooperation and a solid front among employers and unions is needed to calm unreasonable fears about the disease in the workplace.

AIDS Policy in Government Agencies AIDS policy approaches in government agencies tend (a) to not exist or (b) to follow one of the corporate models. A good example of an AIDS-specific government policy is the statement issued by the New York Governor's Office of Employee Relations in 1987. Entitled "Employment Issues Related to AIDS," the five-page statement advises all New York State departments and agencies that

> Persons with clinically defined AIDS or other HIV-related conditions are often well enough to participate in everyday activities, including employment, during subacute phases of the illness. There is no evidence that the disease has been transmitted in the workplace environment through casual contact. Laboratory and epidemiologic data have consistently demonstrated that transmission of the HIV virus, and hence increased risk of AIDS, has been limited to cases where there has been a direct transfer of infected blood or semen. Studies of family members of persons with AIDS, and of health care workers dealing with AIDS patients, have not demonstrated infection by the HIV virus by any other means of transmission.
>
> Based on the best scientific evidence and judgment currently available, no restrictions should be placed on the employment of persons with AIDS, AIDS-related complex (ARC) or a positive HIV antibody blood test, if their health status enables them to perform the duties required by their positions. There is no scientific or medical justification for testing employees for the sole purpose of assessing prospective or current employability.

The rest of the statement covers common questions and answers about AIDS, AIDS transmission and AIDS in the workplace. For example, it is suggested that rumors about an employee having

AIDS should be treated "as you would any other rumor that may be disruptive to workplace operations. Deal with the source of the rumor, if known, and take steps to stop it." Supervisors are warned to maintain confidentiality of medical information about employees, and are advised that the New York State Division of Human Rights has ruled that AIDS is considered a medical condition falling within the protected definition of a disability under the Human Rights Law.

The New York policy statement concludes with the observation that

> Underlying all of this advice [to managers and employee relations officers] must be the basic human understanding that a person with AIDS is ill, possibly very ill, and is entitled to humane treatment. It is our responsibility to deal with this problem in the most compassionate way possible, balancing this within the broader context of a human resources management approach which assures a minimum of disruption in the work of the State which needs to be accomplished.

Advantages/Disadvantages of Choice of Policy Approach

The choice of policy approach must relate to corporate style and to a rational analysis of what is likely to be most successful in a given workplace environment. Doing nothing, not deciding, are rarely successful approaches. The critical question will be how well your task force has faced the relevant issues and made the necessary decisions in good faith, without shirking its responsibility.

The "life-threatening illness" approach offers the advantage of practicing what you preach when you say there is no fundamental reason to treat AIDS differently from other major illnesses. It avoids suggestions of discrimination in favor of AIDS while it includes major health issues of potential interest and concern to every employee. The topic of catastrophic illness is currently receiving considerable media and political attention. Every employee or insured dependent under the organization's health plan is at least potentially at risk for cancer, stroke or heart disease. A life-threatening illness policy has the widest application and is useful for non–AIDS-related purposes. It is thus far the most widely accepted approach in the business community.

An "AIDS-specific" policy acknowledges the potential impact of this new epidemic in the workplace, squarely addresses the issue, lets employees know very clearly where the organization stands, and is in itself an important document in an educational program about the disease. If an AIDS-specific policy is selected, it should also address other life-threatening illnesses, in effect, becoming the mirror image of the life-threatening illness approach, with the emphasis merely reversed. The only disadvantage of an AIDS-specific policy may be that other life-threatening illnesses, which frankly will be far more common in the workplace than AIDS, are not specifically mentioned.

The "no-policy" policy works well for the few organizations whose point of view about AIDS is clearly communicated to the employees. Successful use of this approach may require major organization-wide education programs as a companion piece. The disadvantage of the no-policy approach is that it may indicate that the company is avoiding any choice at all. A successful no-policy policy requires a great deal of integrity on the part of management.

Policy Development as an Educational Experience

Whether your company chooses a life-threatening illness policy, an AIDS-specific policy, or a no-policy policy is not the critical issue. What is important is that the policy development process become an opportunity to face the issues and educate employers and other stakeholders within your organization, including top management, about AIDS. As the human resources director of one large public transportation system reported, "working through the internal review and approval process for a position or policy statement regarding AIDS/ARC is an important educational process. It also takes time." It is vital that the policy choice, whatever it may be, have the necessary support within your organization to make it work, whatever that may mean in the context of your workplace.

Any approach to AIDS in the workplace requires education about the disease and about the social and political issues that surround it. The policy development process is a superb opportunity for educating key managers and important opinion makers within your organization. The task force should remain keenly aware of both its opportunities and its responsibilities around the matter of education.

Plan Communication About AIDS

Once you have established an organizational point of view about AIDS and have chosen a policy approach, it is necessary to decide when, how and by whom that information will be circulated in your organization. As is the case with every other aspect of AIDS, your own organizational structure, size and style will determine to whom you need to communicate with about AIDS, and how and when that communication should take place. By this point, there should have already been extensive communication among the members of the planning task force and with top management about fundamental AIDS-related matters.

The purpose of this planning exercise is to prepare your organization to deal calmly and rationally with an actual or rumored case of AIDS within your workforce. That goal cannot be achieved if all the information about AIDS remains a classified secret limited to a few people. Your task force needs to determine who within your organization should have and understand the information, if the goal of managing AIDS on the job is to be achieved.

Every employee, without exception, could benefit from information about AIDS. At a minimum, staff people and key managers who would be called upon to participate in handling an actual case of AIDS or in advising line managers how to handle an actual case should be included in the communication. The shape and size of this minimum group would depend on how your company is organized and how the various staff departments and line functions interact.

Key people within the human resources, employee assistance, legal and medical departments would undoubtedly be among the first contacted if an AIDS crisis occurs. Line supervisors and their managers are likely to be contacted as an inquiry goes up the chain of command; they need to be included in the communication. Whoever is likely to be called upon for information, advice or a decision in an actual case of AIDS needs to be included now so they will be prepared, informed and able to react appropriately when the time comes. Identify those people within your organization, list them, and plan the process of briefing them about AIDS and about your organization's planned response to it.

Prepare Now for Crisis Management

Since a poorly managed AIDS crisis represents potential harm to your organization, it is useful at this stage to plan out how you would manage a crisis, should one occur, and work backwards from there to who needs to be prepared about AIDS. Given the way your organization functions when it functions best, consider how a personnel or labor crisis situation would be handled. Again, consider what you already know how to do, and how your own organizational culture functions.

The natural flow of communication or of requests for assistance and advice may vary depending on where the crisis first erupts. It is important to work through several scenarios to determine who the players would be under varying circumstances. It is important, however, that you exercise caution in making projections as to where AIDS might show up in your organization based on stereotypical assumptions about who is most likely to get AIDS, and who is not likely to get AIDS. Your assumptions will very likely be wrong.

AIDS can show up anywhere, within the brawniest hard-hat occupations, in the executive suite or anywhere else. Companies with extensive experience with this disease have found that AIDS appears within any occupation, in the factory or in the office, among line or staff, exempt or nonexempt, union or nonunion positions. Persons who perform manual labor are no more or less likely to get AIDS than those who perform management functions. It would be a mistake to make assumptions about where AIDS might or might not strike based on guesswork as to who is likely to get AIDS.

Prepare Line Supervisors

The line supervisors who directly supervise the employees of your organization are the people who first will confront whatever crisis occurs about AIDS on the job. They need to know what to do. They need to be prepared. They need to be included in an educational process about AIDS now.

Organizations frequently educate staff employees about AIDS, preparing the human resources people first and then others who would perform advisory roles during an AIDS crisis. Too often, the frontline supervisors, those who directly can do the most good and the most harm, are left out until it is too late. Educating staff people can be a useless exercise if the line personnel don't know to call on them for assistance about this issue. Whether or not you should include every supervisor in an education process depends, again, on the specifics of your organizational structure and style. But widespread inclusion of line supervisors is the best insurance against a poorly managed crisis.

Bear in mind that when your task force considers the issue of how far down the line to carry out a basic educational effort, all of the fear and discomfort and resistance will come up again, and tend to restrict communication about your point of view and policy about AIDS. Remain aware of your own psychological resistance to dealing with the issue. It's easy to want to keep this issue "in the closet," in the task force or among the top staff.

To achieve the benefits of the planning you have done, however, requires that you involve those who will be called on first to face irrational or angry workers, and who immediately must have basic information about the issue and the organization's response to it. They need to know what this issue is about, who they can call on for help and information. They need to know how decisions will be made, even what kinds of decisions can be made under different circumstances. They need to know enough to feel confident of their ability, with upper management's support, to resolve a crisis in a way that complies with the law and works for the employees they have to supervise day after day after day.

Review the Elements of a Planned Approach

As a guide to help you review and chart your progress, we summarize here the elements of a planned approach to AIDS, as contrasted with an unplanned and reactive approach. A planned approach requires five strategic steps. The first two steps are: (1) develop a point of view about AIDS; (2) decide whether to have a policy about AIDS and determine what that policy will be.

The next two steps go beyond the individuals involved in the initial planning process elements and deal with (3) communicating within the organization about your organization's point of view and policy about AIDS; and (4) educating employees about AIDS. These two steps in the process, then, require planning for communication about AIDS in the workplace. As part of planning for communication, you need to consider the fifth step of a planned approach to AIDS in the workplace: (5) develop a contingency plan for AIDS crisis management and determine how planned crisis management relates to communication in general.

Every employee should be provided with some minimum information about AIDS and about how your organization plans to handle it. Ideally, all employees would receive information that would allow them to avoid any AIDS risk off the job, information they could pass to their family and especially their teenage children.

At the other end of the spectrum, at least key staff and line management people must be fully informed about what the disease is, what its implications are for the workplace, how to educate others about it and how the organization would respond to it. It is also recommended that all line supervisors be included in the initial educational process about the workplace aspects of AIDS. They are the people who will be called on to handle a crisis if one develops; they are the people whose judgment on the spot will become either the basis of or defense against any future litigation.

5 ‖ Designing and Implementing AIDS Education Programs

The task force has made a decision to educate the workforce about AIDS. The same advice that applies to planning for AIDS applies to AIDS education: (1) Deal with AIDS, or education about AIDS, the same way you would deal with any other workplace issue; (2) do what you already know how to do; and (3) be consistent with your own organizational culture and style.

Every company already has a variety of established procedures and channels of communication for educating employees about a myriad of issues in the workplace. Those same procedures and channels of communication should be used to inform employees about AIDS. Review your organization's methods of communicating with employees and list the options. Be aware of how your employees respond to various existing channels of communication and pick what works best for your situation.

Published materials are necessary components of any education program; however, there is no substitute for an in-person presentation of the facts about AIDS with an opportunity for employees to ask questions. Nothing is quite so effective as a competent and informed speaker looking an employee in the eye and saying "you're not at risk for AIDS at work," and then proceeding to deal calmly and fairly with that employee's specific concerns and questions. So it may not be enough to hand every employee a brochure or pamphlet about AIDS.

The best AIDS education program requires the personal involvement of management and employees. For many people AIDS is a highly personal issue. A variety of methods will be required to effectively reach all employees, but provision should be made for face-to-face presentations for some employees. The experience of many organizations confirms that the in-person small group presentation is the most effective way to educate employees about AIDS and to resolve individual fears and concerns.

Some organizations, Bank of America, for example, argue that since they do not have small group, companywide sessions for all employees on other human resources issues, they need not hold such sessions for AIDS education. Instead, they prefer to use the small group process more selectively for certain employees, or when the situation in a specific work unit demands it. This is a defendable position, especially for large workforces.

On the other hand, Levi Strauss began a process in 1987 by which they present AIDS information in small groups to their entire U.S. workforce. To our knowledge, they are the first Fortune 500 company to present AIDS education in the small group format to all of their employees in this country. A feature of their educational program is a videotape prepared especially for their employees.

We strongly suggest that managers and line supervisors be given the advantage of the small group approach. Managers and line supervisors play a vital role in the management of AIDS issues. If they mismanage a crisis, the damage can be considerable. Therefore, the small group procedure is a valuable investment for these important employees.

Getting Started

One way to initiate an employee education program is to publish an article about AIDS in the company newsletter. This establishes the topic of AIDS as a legitimate concern to the company and its employees. Another approach is to purchase or prepare a simple pamphlet about AIDS to be distributed at work or mailed to employees at their homes. New England Bell Telephone Co. recently took this approach. Bear in mind that family reactions and fears influence the employee's reactions and fears. It is a good idea to include the family members in distribution of AIDS materials.

If your company uses videotape education programs, a videotape about AIDS could be purchased or developed in-house and distributed through your normal channels for video materials. A number of companies have found videotapes quite effective, including Potomac Electric Power Company in Washington, D.C., California's Pacific Bell Telephone, Pennsylvania's Westinghouse and Southern Company Services of Atlanta. Companies that typically use posters about health issues may find it useful to purchase or prepare informational posters about AIDS. Companies that sponsor forums or bring in speakers about health topics should do the same with AIDS. Organizations that have established channels for distributing information promoting employee health could use the same channels to communicate about AIDS.

Numerous companies have made information available through employee assistance or medical departments. At companies with strong medical departments, such as Westinghouse or Pacific Bell Telephone, the medical unit originally took the leadership position about AIDS. At companies like Levi Strauss, Wells Fargo Bank, and Pacific Gas & Electric, employee assistance departments have primary responsibility for the AIDS issue. In a variation on this approach, Crowley Maritime Corporation has assigned AIDS education responsibility to its circuit-riding employee assistance manager, who regularly visits the company's far-flung locations on three coasts and who disseminates AIDS information as part of his rounds. Interest in AIDS has become great enough in a few large organizations that they have set up 800-number hotlines to provide information to workers about AIDS, either as it impacts the workplace or as a means by which employees can get information about personal risk off the job.

It is worth noting that patterns of shifting employee interest in the topic of AIDS are now fairly predictable over time. Initial employee interest in the subject nearly always focuses on fears about personal safety in the workplace: Can I get AIDS at work? What are my risks at work or in other aspects of my life? Once these initial concerns about casual contagion are satisfied, employee interest ultimately shifts to sexual matters: Am I at risk for AIDS because of some incident in my sexual past? How can I manage my dating relationships to avoid AIDS? What should I tell my adolescent children about sex and AIDS? Employers should be prepared for this shift in interest after the initial concerns about workplace exposure are satisfied.

There is no single "right way" to educate employees about AIDS. A number of different approaches repeated over time are needed to get the information across accurately. AIDS education is a process, not an event. Some of your employees may be at risk and will need a different level of information than those who are not. Your education programs should be designed to accommodate different needs within your workforce.

Unfortunately, the AIDS epidemic will be with us for many more years. It will be an ongoing topic of interest in the press and in the political arena, and it will be an ongoing long-term issue for organizations of all kinds. Ongoing educational programs will be necessary, and over time all available channels of communication with employees will have to be used at one time or another.

Face-to-Face Communication: Small Group Presentations

Ultimately you need to prepare for facilitated informational sessions with groups of employees, the in-person, face-to-face communication about this topic where the opportunity exists to freely ask questions. We recommend that in-person group informational sessions form the core of the AIDS education program.

The most effective AIDS educational sessions require meetings with groups of employees, led by a trained and informed speaker who can present the basic information about the disease, explain what the company is going to do about it and answer employee questions clearly and comfortably. The size of the group will depend in part on the talent and personality of the speaker. We have seen groups of 100 or more people effectively discuss the issue. More typically, though, groups of twenty-five or so are more manageable, and allow people more freedom to ask personal questions.

Small groups have a variety of advantages for educational purposes:

- Small group interaction in work settings is fairly common, so people are used to it.

- Small groups allow people to interact, discuss and ask questions, which maximizes integration of learning.

- Employees feel less threatened in a small group of their peers and can engage the subject more freely; that is, they feel safer, especially where the topic may be an awkward one.

- A small group is easier for most group leaders to work with.

- More can be accomplished in less time than with larger groups.

- It is usually more practical and efficient to gather a small group of people together from a particular work unit to conduct a short meeting than to gather a much larger group for a longer period of time.

Agenda for the Group Sessions

While the presentation must be appropriate to the specific audience, there are several elements that should be included in any employee group presentation about AIDS.

1. The leader should explain why the organization has decided to deal with AIDS. This creates the context for what follows. AIDS is now a business issue. Exactly what you say will depend on the audience.
   a. If the audience is senior management, the discussion will focus on the business reasons for dealing with AIDS.
   b. If the audience is line supervisors, the discussion will focus on the increasing likelihood that they will be approached by concerned employees, so they need to be informed about both the disease and the company's response to it; they also need to be prepared to deal with rumors and employee fears.
   c. If the audience is line employees, the discussion will focus on providing information about AIDS so that they will feel safe in the workplace, to let them know there are additional channels of information and counseling available should they become concerned.

2. The leader should explain the organization's position about employees with AIDS. (In initial presentations to senior management, this may not be a part of your introduction since the company position may not have been established, but options and recommendations can be presented.) The company's official position on AIDS establishes the context in which the overall issue of AIDS can be discussed and puts management's stamp of approval on the factual point of view about the disease. The company's position is a statement that "we have checked this out and this is the truth regarding AIDS." The company's credibility stands behind the presentation of information and suggests what kinds of attitudes about AIDS are expected of employees once the facts are explained.

3. The leader should present information about AIDS simply and clearly. A handout or employee brochure with the basic facts can be distributed. Employees are generally not familiar with medical terminology nor comfortable with medical explanations

of complicated diseases. They want to know if they can get AIDS at work, and if not, why not. This information should include an explanation of how AIDS is and is not transmitted, stressing the fact that AIDS cannot be transmitted by nonsexual contact at work.

4. The leader may use an educational videotape to clarify and back up the factual presentation. A highly recommended video for this purpose is "An Epidemic of Fear—AIDS in the Workplace," an award-winning program originally commissioned by the Business Leadership Task Force of the Bay Area and jointly updated in late 1987 by Wells Fargo Bank, Pacific Bell, Chevron Corporation, BankAmerica Foundation, Pacific Gas and Electric, McKesson Foundation, Blue Shield of California, and Fireman's Fund Insurance Company.

5. The leader should hold a question and answer session as the final segment of the group meeting. Questions should be encouraged; employees should understand that there are no dumb questions about AIDS, that questions on the mind of one person are likely to be on the minds of others and that asking the question serves everyone's interests. It is important that people be encouraged to freely express their concerns. The facilitator needs to be a skilled listener, because the "real" question may be concealed by the more obvious question being asked. The question and answer session is the best test of the facilitator's communication skills.

Generally, an educational group session containing these elements will require a minimum of one hour, and up to 90 minutes is sometimes preferable. The time breakdown would be (a) five to ten minutes on why we are dealing with AIDS and what the company's point of view is; (b) 15 to 20 minutes on the facts about AIDS; (c) 25 minutes for a videotape about AIDS; and (d) at least 15 minutes for questions, depending on audience interest.

As is the case with any other topic, the content of the presentation must be appropriate to the audience. A presentation about AIDS to human relations personnel or to senior managers may well be quite different in content and style than a presentation to factory workers. It is also important that the presenter be appropriate for the specific audience and be able to establish a rapport with them. A relationship of trust and confidence between the presenter and the audience is essential.

Consistent with the concept of audience credibility, a joint presentation by the company and the appropriate labor unions may in many cases be advantageous. In our experience, labor unions have been extremely helpful with AIDS education programs and with the development of policies about AIDS in the workplace. Many unions were pioneers in the initiation of workplace policies about AIDS that later came to be adopted by management. Union participation in employee education programs about AIDS should not be overlooked, and should in fact be encouraged.

Mandatory or Voluntary Sessions

Most employee educational sessions about other work-related matters are not voluntary; attendance is expected as part of the job. The same approach should be taken with AIDS education. The company wants all appropriate employees to have this information; there are sound business reasons for wanting them to have it, as well as business risks to be incurred if employees do not have this information.

The experience of companies who have tried voluntary sessions is that employees are sometimes reluctant to attend because their presence at such a meeting might be considered a "statement" that they have some special reason to be interested in the topic. Employees who are genuinely interested in learning about AIDS might nevertheless stay away because of concern about "what others will think." Do what you would normally do about attendance at employee education programs of business importance—get them there. The employees most likely to avoid these sessions are also the people most likely to become the source of problems later on.

Locate Educational Resources and Speakers

In the beginning you will likely need outside assistance to help you get started, to educate yourselves, to have your own questions and concerns answered, and perhaps even to help deal with top management. How to locate educational resources, speakers and consultants will depend a great deal on where you are located. Those companies in major cities will have an easier time finding a consultant than those located in less-populated areas.

The metropolitan areas hit hardest by AIDS all have local AIDS organizations whose role includes dissemination of information about the disease. These organizations are quite willing to cooperate with employer programs about AIDS in the workplace. Morrison & Foerster, a major law firm, was able to obtain volunteer speakers from AIDS agencies in the several cities in which the firm operates. The speakers were well qualified, and the cost was simply a donation to the sponsoring organizations. (See the Resource Section in the Appendix for the name of an AIDS organization near you.)

There is likely to be at least one hospital in your community that has become the central hospital for AIDS patients. Call that hospital and speak with the infection control nurse. Infection control nurses in significant hospitals tend to be knowledgeable about AIDS. It is their job to know how diseases are transmitted and to educate the nursing and medical staff of their hospitals about disease prevention. Ask the nurse for advice about speakers; perhaps she or he would be willing to speak to your task force, human resources people or even groups of employees. Like most professionals who deal with AIDS, infection control nurses tend to be helpful to organizations conducting education about this disease.

Most state health departments and many larger local city/county health departments have assigned specific personnel to deal with

AIDS-related matters. Call your health department, ask for the AIDS unit—or in the absence of one, the infectious disease unit. Explain your needs and ask for their advice and help. Public information about AIDS is a formal responsibility of health departments; it is their job to help you in educating your workforce.

Contact the state and local medical societies. Ask for the names of knowledgeable and effective speakers who can discuss AIDS with the general public. Occupational disease units within hospitals or medical schools generally have staff who are familiar with AIDS issues in the workplace. Medical schools almost always employ experts who track the latest information about AIDS; they may not always be good educators for lay audiences, however, so you'll have to make your own determination of their appropriateness for your educational program. Local Chambers of Commerce also may have information about potential local speakers on AIDS in the workplace. Professional organizations such as the American Society for Training and Development, and the North American Congress on Employee Assistance Programs, and the American Occupational Health Association have seminars and speakers on the subject of AIDS in the workplace at their national conferences.

Finally, talk with human resources, employee assistance, medical, legal, training and employee communications people from other companies. Those with AIDS' experience are usually quite willing to share what they have learned. You may find other companies in your region or within your industry that have already been through the basics about AIDS and will pass on what they have learned. Inter-company cooperation has been a hallmark of the corporate response to AIDS in this country.

A Word of Caution About Using Your Regular Physicians Many employers have existing professional relationships with physicians or group medical practices and may be tempted to call on them for assistance about AIDS. A word of caution is in order. AIDS is still a relatively new issue. The typical general practitioner knows little, if anything, about AIDS and may in fact have more misinformation about the disease than the least informed of your employees. Some physicians know little more than what they see on television, although people assume that physicians always know what they are talking about. The assumption can be disastrous. Inaccurate information from an uninformed physician can cause untold damage to the best educational program.

If you are going to ask a private physician to consult with your company about AIDS, you must determine for yourself whether that individual is qualified to do so. Ask questions, and listen carefully to the answers. Compare what you're hearing, the attitudes and points of view being expressed, with information from the Surgeon General, the Centers for Disease Control, and other business organizations and labor unions. Understand that a medical degree is no assurance of knowledge about AIDS, and is even less assurance of the holder's ability to effectively communicate to laymen about AIDS. Many doctors, while superb clinicians, are poor educators, incapable of communicating in layman's terms. Your responsibility is to judge whether a physician will be an asset or a liability to your AIDS education program.

Select Internal AIDS Resource People

At some point, you may want to train in-house AIDS resource people who are knowledgeable about the epidemic, capable both of counseling individuals and making group presentations about AIDS, and who can assist with conflict resolution should it become necessary. Many larger organizations have found that having AIDS resource people within the organization is helpful. The advantages of having in-house expertise available are fairly obvious. With in-house people, they are part of the organization, familiar with its structure, culture and style of communication. As insiders, they are perceived as being "one of us" and therefore more trustworthy. They have a vested interest in the well-being of the organization and its workforce.

Many organizations with on-going AIDS education programs have trained individual staff members to be internal AIDS educators. These people are usually drawn from the employee assistance, human resources, health promotion, affirmative action or equal employment departments. It is not the function of these resource people to become medical experts on AIDS or to devote full-time to AIDS issues. Rather, their role is to make presentations about the disease, explain the company's policy about AIDS, and be able to answer questions or refer people to appropriate sources of information or services.

Internal AIDS educators or resource people need not be medical specialists. Some of the finest early pioneers in the field of AIDS in the workplace, Brian Lawton at Wells Fargo, Nancy Merrit and Kathy Armstrong at Bank of America, Michael Eriksen, Susan Walters and Steve Coulter at Pacific Bell, Yvonne Ellison-Sandler at Levi Strauss, and Gerry Hughes at Chevron are not medical specialists. They all had other functions within their organizations, but they were willing to learn and were not intimidated by medical jargon and scientific information. They also were good listeners and skilled communicators, had good human relations skills, and were keenly interested in the subject. In short, they had the needed qualifications to become good AIDS resources.

The most essential skill needed to be an AIDS resource person is the ability to assist people in discussing their fears and to guide them towards authoritative sources for answers to their questions. Resource people also need to have dealt with their own issues about AIDS, sex or drugs so that their personal biases will not affect their interactions with employees. Resource people need to understand and deal with the occasional hostile reaction; they need to be patient people. Finally, they need to serve as role models at work for employee responses to the AIDS issue.

The following description developed for Syntex may be useful to your organization as a guide to the role of the internal AIDS resource:

An AIDS Resource is someone who is identified in the workplace as the person to go to for information about AIDS. An AIDS Resource is not an AIDS expert. He or she is sensitive to the human relations issues, and legal issues, and employee concerns about the disease, understands and can discuss the company's position on illness in the workplace, knows company policy and how to interpret that policy as it relates to illness in the workplace, and has the latest and most up-to-date resource materials on AIDS.

As an AIDS Resource, you will be often asked questions about the medical aspects of AIDS, including antibody testing, symptoms, treatments, diagnosis, who to see for medical evaluation. Because you are not a medical expert, it's always advisable to decline to answer purely medical questions, to decline to offer medical opinions or advice, and to refer such questions to appropriate medical personnel. Your job is to be able to understandably communicate the basic facts about AIDS—which are available through the Surgeon General's report, numerous pamphlets, publications, hotlines, and from this book—and to know where to refer people for further information.

An important part of being an AIDS Resource is to be an example, or role model, to others concerning the human and emotional issues surrounding this unfortunate disease. There is considerable fear and misunderstanding about AIDS. People often have too little information, incomplete information, or in some cases, so much information that they suffer from "information overload" and can't sort out the facts. They often remember news reports of speculation and rumor about AIDS equally with pieces of facts about AIDS.

Beyond the basic facts about transmission, which are pretty clear and fairly easy to explain at this point, most employees are not interested in, and are often confused by, the medical aspects of AIDS. They often simply need a forum in which to deal with their concerns and with other personal issues surrounding AIDS. Therefore, medical expertise is not necessary, and often not even desired, in employee AIDS education programs or in AIDS Resource people.

How many AIDS Resource people your organization needs depends on the size and distribution of your workforce, and the degree of impact of the epidemic in the geographic areas in which you operate. Rarely will these be full-time positions; they are part-time additional duties for existing personnel. A highly decentralized and widely distributed organization may require a number of such people.

Train Your Resource People

Use outside experts and educational consultants to help educate and train your internal AIDS resource people. Send them to seminars on AIDS in the workplace being sponsored by professional and trade associations and by business consulting firms. Provide your resource people with the latest pamphlets, videotapes and textbooks. Advise them to keep up with newspaper and magazine articles on AIDS: *Business Week, U.S. News*, the *Wall Street Journal* and other more specialized publications like the *Arbitration Journal, Personnel Journal*, the *Legal Administrator, Psychology Today* and *AIDS and the Law* frequently publish articles on AIDS.

If your organization has videotape facilities, tape your resource people practicing presentations and answering questions about AIDS. Let other resource people comment and share reactions in a group setting, using a review of the tapes for instructional feedback. Use whatever techniques and in-house resources you have available for staff training and development.

Locate Useful Pamphlets and Videotapes

One task of AIDS resource people is to keep up with available instructional materials. The supply and variety of such materials increases daily. Among the best pamphlets currently available about AIDS in the workplace are these:

1. "AIDS in the Workplace, a Guide for Employees" is a concise, to-the-point handout about AIDS for workers. This pamphlet

was commissioned as part of the San Francisco Business Leadership Task Force AIDS package. Marketing rights to the publication, like those to the accompanying videotape ("An Epidemic of Fear—AIDS in the Workplace"), were donated by the participating companies to the San Francisco AIDS Foundation. Proceeds from the sale of these corporate-generated materials support the ongoing work of the foundation. Single copy or bulk orders of the brochure and copies of the videotape (VHS, Beta or 3/4 inch) are available from the foundation's Marketing Department, 333 Valencia Street, 4th Floor, San Francisco, CA 94103; telephone (415) 861-3397.

2. The Surgeon General's Report on AIDS (see Appendix) is hard to beat for clarity, completeness and appropriateness for all audiences. Copies can be ordered from the local office of the U.S. Public Health Service (check the phone listings under U.S. government agencies) or the U.S. Public Health Service, Public Affairs Office, 725-H Hubert H. Humphrey Building, 200 Independence Avenue, SW, Washington, D.C. 20201; telephone (202) 245-6867.

3. A superb labor union publication is "The AIDS Book, Information for Workers" by the Service Employees International Union, AFL-CIO, 1313 L Street, NW, Washington, D.C. 20005; telephone (202) 898-3200.

4. The American Red Cross has published videotapes and print materials about AIDS. The Red Cross has a great deal of credibility with employees. Contact the local Red Cross chapter or the American Red Cross AIDS Education Office, 1730 D Street, NW, Washington, D.C. 20006; telephone (202) 737-8300.

5. The San Francisco AIDS Foundation publishes a catalog of AIDS educational materials. It is probably the most complete resource guide to print and videotape materials. The catalog is updated quarterly and is free upon request. Contact the foundation at

333 Valencia Street, 4th Floor, San Francisco, CA 94103; telephone (415) 861-3397.

Understand That For Some Employees, Education May Not Be Enough

While AIDS education programs generally accomplish what they set out to do, there are always a few people who can't get the message. "There is something about the topic of AIDS that can cause some otherwise intelligent and rational people to completely lose their basic common sense" explains AIDS educator Pat Christen of the San Francisco AIDS Foundation. AIDS educators regularly report that a few employees remain hysterically fearful about this disease, even after all the facts, all the medical evidence, all the considered weight of scientific opinion confirm that people aren't being exposed simply by being around someone who has the disease. Understanding this occasional irrationality is an important part of managing AIDS in the workplace. It is important that AIDS resource people understand the psychological mechanism involved, which we have labeled AIDS Fear Syndrome. It typically is experienced by only a small—but sometimes noisy—minority of any given workplace audience. For such people, overreactive fear of AIDS seems to be based on the *interactions* of two separate psychological mechanisms:

1. A gut-level fear reaction that comes out of a basic survival instinct and which operates independently of the intellect. In its simplest form, it is often referred to as "fear of the unknown."

2. A blind rejection of AIDS because of the people who have it, due to a deep-seated and only partially conscious negative indoctrination about sex and homosexuality. Let's consider each of these mechanisms individually and then see how they operate together.

Our experience with AIDS Fear Syndrome confirms that people have a remarkable protective capability to avoid, almost instinctively, the possibility of exposure to infectious disease. At a deep, instinctual level our minds can send us a compelling "danger signal" to quickly move out of harm's way. This instinctive reaction is independent of our intellect; the reaction does not depend on knowledge or intellectual assessment of risk.

It is our *instinct's* job to move us away from danger; it is our *intellect's* job to evaluate the danger rationally, and to make decisions and choices about the reality of danger. The instinctive warning doesn't evaluate the facts; it simply warns in a way that we cannot ignore.

A part of AIDS Fear Syndrome comes from our natural protective instincts. The other part of the syndrome comes from social conditioning about homosexuality, venereal disease, drugs and sex. Most people have been conditioned from earliest childhood to fear and have extremely negative views about homosexuals and homosexuality. Some people are even taught to hate homosexuals and to fear being in their presence. On a day-to-day basis, most people are not aware of these feelings. Venereal disease also elicits strong negative feelings. People are taught that venereal diseases are nasty and disgusting. People are taught about the evils of drug use and sexual promiscuity. In short, in our culture large numbers of people have been negatively conditioned about the very issues that have become associated with AIDS and the AIDS epidemic. For many people, guilt about their own sexual behavior or fantasies may complicate the problem. Their minds associate AIDS with the strong negative feelings and fears that are attached to the other issues, without their necessarily understanding why. To make matters worse this lack of understanding of their own emotional reactions tends to compound them, making them stronger and less manageable. As a consequence, excessive fear reactions to AIDS have little to do with AIDS as a disease, but are caused by the triggering of old and often unconscious emotions.

When these strong, culturally acquired feelings are *combined* with the instinctive fear reactions about diseases in general, what can result is a strong combination of fear, anger, irrationality and an unwillingness to hear or understand the facts. The resource person will discover that typically people want to avoid dealing with these emotionally charged issues by "pushing away" the issues, *and* the person or persons they deem to be the source of their negative feelings, and *find a socially acceptable reason for doing so*. The socially acceptable reason is usually based on religious or moral beliefs.

Virtually everyone will experience some degree of AIDS fear upon their first face-to-face encounter with this new disease. We had that experience, as did most of those now responsible for corporate AIDS policies. For some, the initial response is a mild fear reaction; it passes quickly. For others, the reaction will be stronger and longer lasting. Time, patience and the repetitive presentation of the facts about AIDS will eventually solve the problem for all but the most recalcitrant.

Dr. Constance Wofsy, Co-Director of the AIDS Clinic at San Francisco General Hospital and an AIDS educator, makes an insightful comment in the videotape "An Epidemic of Fear—AIDS in the Workplace" that is worth repeating here:

> Information about AIDS isn't heard with just one go-round.
> The first go-round leads to fear and denial.
> The second go-round leads to accepting that maybe this is something I'm going to have to know about.
> The third go-round leads to a little bit of intellectual curiosity, because it really is kind of an interesting topic.
> The fourth go-round tends to lead to real interest.
> The fifth go-round usually puts people in a place where they finally become a little bit more concerned about the other person than themselves.
> And you have to go through it all of those times for everyone.

Educational programs should concentrate on the facts about AIDS, rather than attempt to change deep-seated cultural beliefs or religious conditioning. What usually happens for people holding strong beliefs is that they eventually are able to *separate* their beliefs about the people who get AIDS and the way AIDS is spread from the facts about AIDS transmission at work. They eventually realize that it is okay for them to disapprove of many of the people who get AIDS and of how AIDS is spread, but still understand that they are not at risk simply because of the presence of a co-worker who has the disease. AIDS Fear Syndrome is generally "curable."

Manage a Crisis About AIDS at Work

If a crisis develops in a work unit over a real or rumored case of AIDS, special handling is required, as it would be for a workplace crisis of any sort. Crises are characterized by anger, miscommunications, defending of positions and unwillingness to listen. Hard feelings may already abound within the work unit over real or imagined grievances. By the time a crisis is declared, the supervisor has already lost control of the situation, and outside help is needed.

The immediate goal of crisis intervention is to calm the situation and gain time to learn what has happened, to identify the issues and to work out a solution. Longer-term solutions would include restoring the damaged relationships within the unit so that there is a return to normal working conditions.

Crisis resolution may require the intervention and assistance of two people from outside the troubled department. First, there should be an AIDS resource person who can intelligently and calmly address the medical/factual side of a controversy, answer questions and generally exert a calming effect on the situation. Second, there should be a person, perhaps the supervisor's boss or the person ultimately responsible for the unit, such as a production supervisor or plant manager, who can speak for the company about the policy and labor relations issues that are a part of the controversy. In other words, it is important to keep the AIDS facts separate from management policy or labor relations issues.

In many cases involving AIDS crises, non-AIDS issues are found to be an underlying part of the conflict. The presence on the job of an AIDS patient, real or imagined, may well trigger unresolved conflicts: preexisting anger at the ill employee himself or herself; anger at the supervisor for being insensitive to employee concerns; anger at the company about other employment policies, such as affirmative action, from which "advantages" are given to minorities or the handicapped; or policies that favor such groups over "ordinary" employees. Those purely employee–employer labor relations issues have nothing to do with AIDS, but will be a part of the crisis that must be addressed. Keeping the AIDS issues separate from the labor relations issues and having the employees recognize them as separate issues is extremely useful to a resolution of the conflict. The AIDS resource person should address only issues relating to AIDS; the personnel or management person should address the issues relating to other matters.

The small group session with ten to fifteen people is best for conflict resolution. It is vital that people have a chance to fully communicate what is on their minds, and to have their communication heard by management without being summarily dismissed or prejudged. They may have legitimate complaints. If nothing else, their complaint about working with a person who has AIDS is legitimate if they have had no education about the subject.

If fear of transmission on the job is central to employees' concerns, small group education programs should address their fears. Plenty of time should be allowed for questions, comments and complaints. Full communication is essential to resolve the problem. Although every effort should be made to convince employees that they are not at risk from the presence of an infected co-worker on the job, ultimately it may become obvious that the efforts will not succeed. At that point, it is appropriate for a manager to point out that both company policy and the law support workers with AIDS in continuing to work so long as they're able to do so and that, since there is no medical reason for it to be any other way, the protesting employees are expected to get back to work and return the situation to one of normal business practices. At that point failure to do so would have the same consequences as any other refusal to work without just cause.

Do What You Know How to Do

As we have pointed out, a mistake made by managers is to assume that AIDS is an issue vastly different from other management matters. Every organization routinely communicates with its employees about a variety of topics. The techniques and resources that organizations routinely use for communicating with employees, are available for communicating about AIDS. Properly explained in nonmedical terms, AIDS can be readily understood by both managers and employees. External resources for AIDS education on the job are increasingly available. Internal AIDS resource people can be trained to serve as sources of information, role models and as calming influences should conflict develop. Resources serve as the "people backup" for less personal educational channels, such as corporate newsletters, pamphlets, posters and educational videos.

Those managers who have become practiced at AIDS education at work have learned that it is a personally rewarding experience, communicating with co-workers about a critical matter of general public concern. AIDS resource people have the opportunity to prevent unnecessary conflict, chaos and legal battles on the job over AIDS. They also have the opportunity to actually save the lives of those co-workers whose personal behavior off the job puts them at risk for contracting the disease.

6

A Primer on Prevention: Safe Sex, the Search for a Vaccine and Antibody Testing

As a society, we need to understand that AIDS will be with us for many more years. Our culture, lifestyles and societal points of view, including our business points of view, must adjust to the reality of AIDS for the long haul. A preventive vaccine will eventually be available. A cure is less likely, with the best near-term hope being a drug that could be taken regularly to keep the AIDS virus in check. What all this means is that *prevention* is the key. For those who are not yet infected with this deadly virus, remaining uninfected is very important, and very possible. Informed, responsible, personal action can prevent the transmission of AIDS.

Anyone who has had more than one sex partner in the past several years, or anyone whose current sex partner has had more than one sex partner in the past several years, or anyone who might have a new sex partner in the foreseeable future, needs to know about AIDS prevention. Anyone who might have been exposed to AIDS through a blood transfusion, through artificial insemination with donated sperm, or through blood–clotting medications needs information on AIDS prevention. Anyone who has shared an intravenous drug needle with another person in the past several years, or who might do so even once in the future, or whose sex partner might have done so, needs this information.

If you feel that you don't personally need to know about AIDS prevention, someone close to you may: a co-worker, a friend or relative, an adolescent child. You have the opportunity to help save someone's life by passing on important information. Directly or indirectly, for themselves or others they care about, just about everyone who participates in contemporary life needs to have a basic understanding about AIDS prevention. Because our culture imposes such restrictions on public education about sex, the kind of private, one-on-one educational opportunities that exist among friends and family members become that much more important. Individual participation in AIDS prevention programs will be essential to our ability as a society to stop any further infection by this deadly disease.

As the Surgeon General points out in his report on AIDS,

> Knowing the facts about AIDS can prevent the spread of the disease. Education of those who risk infecting themselves or infecting other people is the only way we can stop the spread of AIDS. The AIDS virus infects only persons who expose themselves to known risk behavior, such as certain types of homosexual and heterosexual sexual activities or the sharing of intravenous drug equipment. In the future AIDS will probably increase and spread among people who are not homosexual or intravenous drug abusers in the same manner as other sexually transmitted diseases like syphilis and gonorrhea.

Four Essential Points About AIDS

Marcia Quackenbush, M.S.W., of the University of California's AIDS Health Project is a nationally respected expert on AIDS education, especially education for parents, teachers and teenagers. What she has learned in educating thousands of people about AIDS applies to all of us. She points out that there are four basic facts about AIDS that everyone needs to understand.

1. AIDS is caused by a virus, not by a lifestyle.
2. AIDS is not casually transmitted.
3. There are circumstances in which AIDS can be transmitted.
4. Preventing the circumstances in which AIDS is transmitted prevents AIDS. AIDS is preventable.

AIDS is caused by a virus, not a lifestyle. If AIDS were caused by a lifestyle, avoiding AIDS would be as simple as avoiding that kind of lifestyle. But AIDS is caused by a virus, a virus that can be spread through certain activities regardless of lifestyle, so preventing AIDS requires learning about, and avoiding, those specific activities. People can engage in a specific lifestyle without spreading AIDS or being at risk for AIDS. The majority of homosexual men in America, for example, have never been infected with the AIDS virus.

Far too many people focus all their attention on the false possibility that AIDS can be acquired just by going through life, by working beside someone who has AIDS, for example, while ignoring the real ways by which AIDS is spread, namely unprotected sexual intercourse or the sharing of unsterilized IV needles. Far too many people have the mistaken idea that AIDS is easy to spread through simple general social or occupational encounters. Far too many people have the very mistaken idea that AIDS is very difficult to spread through heterosexual sex.

It is important to really understand the circumstances under which AIDS can be transmitted. That knowledge, that understanding, could save someone's life—perhaps yours, perhaps someone close to you. For the many people who have absolutely no risk of getting this disease, knowing the circumstances of AIDS transmission will relieve a great deal of anxiety. For the people who could be, or who could become, at risk for AIDS, knowing the circumstances of AIDS transmission will allow them to take appropriate precautions. It is often sadly true that the people who are most concerned about AIDS have no reason to be concerned, while the people who have the most reason to be concerned generally are not concerned enough.

AIDS is preventable. For most of the people who already have AIDS, it may not have been preventable when they first became infected with the virus because the necessary information didn't then exist. Now that information about the AIDS virus exists and is available to anyone who wants it, and now that blood supplies are screened so that there is little risk these days of getting AIDS from a transfusion or from blood-clotting medication, it is fully possible to avoid infection.

Transmission and Prevention

The AIDS virus cannot be passed through the air. The virus cannot penetrate the skin, if picked up on the skin from an environmental surface. It cannot enter the body through the lungs. It cannot be transmitted in food. If the virus is present in the body of someone you know, interactions with that person are safe, unless the interaction makes it possible for the virus to exit the body of the infected person via one of a very few specific body fluids and directly enter the inside of your body.

The Centers for Disease Control identifies AIDS as a blood-borne and sexually transmitted disease. If you have a general understanding of how venereal diseases are transmitted and prevented, you already understand how AIDS is transmitted sexually and how it can be prevented. Sex and IV drug use account for nearly all cases of AIDS. Without those two methods of transmission, there would be no epidemic of AIDS now or in the future. Even with those two methods of transmission, AIDS is preventable.

The AIDS virus is fragile outside the human body and is easily killed by sunlight, common household cleansers or soap and hot water. It needs a moist, temperature-controlled environment in which to survive, and it cannot reproduce by itself the way bacteria do. It also requires a specific point of entry into the human body.

In an infected person, the virus lives in the bloodstream and reproduces inside the T-Helper Cell Lymphocytes that are present in the bloodstream. The virus is found in an infected person's blood. For that reason, direct contact between an infected person's bloodstream and your bloodstream would constitute a danger to you. Two people injecting themselves with a shared and unsterilized needle is an example of dangerous contact and a common way in which AIDS is spread.

Prior to the blood-screening programs instituted in the spring of 1985, it was possible to receive a transfusion of an infected person's blood—another example of a dangerous contact with another person's bloodstream. Blood banks now screen all blood supplies for evidence of AIDS infection and discard any blood found to be infected. The blood supply in major Western countries is now safer than it has ever been.

For health care workers who handle blood supplies as part of their daily routine, the kind of accident in which meaningful quantities of infected blood come into contact with workers' bodies would be a dangerous interaction. Although only a remarkably small number of doctors, nurses and other health care workers have been infected by the AIDS virus at work, large quantities of blood must be handled with caution, and traditional infection control procedures must be followed by all health care workers. Doctors, nurses, lab technicians and orderlies spend their entire working day exposing themselves to blood, feces, urine and vomit and are dramatically more at risk than other kinds of workers. The presence of AIDS doesn't change the basic infection-control rules, but AIDS should provide serious motivation for following them.

Blood-to-blood contact is a method by which several diseases in addition to AIDS, including syphilis and hepatitis, can be transmitted. Sharing needles transmits syphilis, for example. Blood transfusions would transmit syphilis, except that blood-screening programs test all donated blood for evidence of the disease. Nearly one-fourth of all cases of AIDS in America so far have been transmitted by some variation of blood-to-blood contact, mostly from the sharing of unsterilized needles.

Sexual Transmission of AIDS

The Surgeon General and other health authorities remind us that "[AIDS] cannot be spread in the same manner as a common cold or measles or chicken pox. It is contagious in the same way that sexually transmitted diseases, like syphilis and gonorrhea, are contagious." Sexual transmission of the AIDS virus has been responsible for nearly three-fourths of all cases of AIDS reported in the U.S. to date, and probably an even higher percentage elsewhere in the world.

The AIDS virus can be present in the semen of an infected male, or in the vaginal fluids of an infected female. The reason the virus could be in the semen or vaginal fluids is that lymphocytes are present in those fluids. The AIDS virus lives and reproduces in lymphocytes. If a person is infected with the AIDS virus, the virus would be present in their lymphocytes, and the lymphocytes could be in their semen or vaginal fluids. Getting that person's blood, semen or vaginal fluids inside your body would be a dangerous form of interaction, since the person's virus-infected lymphocytes would carry the AIDS virus with them.

Intact human skin is an effective barrier against the AIDS virus. Getting an infected person's blood, semen or vaginal fluid on the outside of your skin would *not* be a dangerous interaction so long as the skin were intact, since the virus cannot penetrate skin. Getting a significant quantity of that person's blood, semen or vaginal fluid onto a large cut or sore on your skin *might* be a dangerous interaction, because, in that case, the opportunity exists for the virus to enter your body and bloodstream. A minimum quantity of the virus would have to actually enter your bloodstream to do any harm, so paper cuts or other small breaks in the skin do not pose a threat. If a cut isn't large or open enough to present an infection problem, requiring a bandage larger than a Band-Aid, it isn't likely to be large or open enough to provide an entry point for the AIDS virus.

Getting an infected person's blood, semen or vaginal fluids onto the *internal* mucous membranes of the body—for example, *inside* the vagina or rectum, or *inside* the urethral canal of the penis— would be a dangerous interaction, since those internal membranes could absorb the virus directly into the bloodstream. The AIDS virus is harmless on the outside of the body, but dangerous on the inside of the body once it gets access to the bloodstream.

Condoms are a key to safe sex. A condom can act as a barrier to prevent semen from entering the body of the receptive partner— male or female. The condom can similarly prevent the penis from directly contacting the vaginal fluids of the woman partner. In laboratory tests conducted in 1985 by AIDS researchers Marc Conant, M.D., and Jay Levy, M.D., it was found that the AIDS virus could *not* penetrate the material of a condom. Condoms have the ability to stop AIDS transmission, just as they can stop syphilis, herpes or gonorrhea.

On the other side of the coin, however, sexually active adults and adolescents almost never receive instruction in the proper use of condoms. Like anything else, condoms can be used improperly; improper use reduces or destroys their effectiveness. Considering how serious are the diseases that condoms are designed to prevent and the number of decades that condoms have been available, it is amazing that almost no information about their proper use has ever been made available. Most of us never took the time or trouble to learn about proper use of condoms; we were too embarrassed to ask or didn't know who to ask, or we had such unpleasant early experiences with condoms that we were anxious to avoid their use under any circumstances.

For those people who have sexual encounters *outside* of long-term fully faithful monogamous relationships, it is time they got serious about condoms and learned how to use them properly. Using condoms properly means using them consistently and without exception. Conversely, consider those couples who have been totally faithful to one another since before 1977 when the AIDS virus first arrived in America. Unless there is danger that one or both partners might become infected through some other method (such as a blood transfusion), the use of a condom is unnecessary.

The AIDS virus has also been found occasionally in minute quantities in the saliva and tears of some infected persons. One would need a quart of saliva or tears to become infected, and then it would be necessary to find a way to get the fluids into the bloodstream so that the viruses could find lymphocytes to infect. While the theoretical risk of "French kissing" has to be conceded as an abstract possibility, there is probably a greater risk of being hit by a falling meteorite than of getting AIDS from French kissing.

The press may still use the euphemism "the exchange of body fluids" when referring to AIDS transmission, but they do so either from unfortunate habit or because they are reluctant to refer to the bodily fluids about which we should really be concerned: blood, semen and vaginal fluids. In all these years, no one has ever contracted AIDS from any bodily fluid other than blood, semen or vaginal secretions.

Risk Groups, Anal Sex and Risk Activities   There is much confusion around the use of the term "risk group." Groups do not spread AIDS. Specific activities spread AIDS. Anyone who engages in those specific activities with an infected person can become infected with the virus, regardless of the gender or sexual orientation of either party. Focusing on the *labels* attached to those who have most commonly gotten AIDS in the past can be misleading to those who engage in the very same activities, but who don't think of themselves as fitting the label. For example, homosexual males are the highest "risk group" for AIDS. Some homosexual males engage in anal intercourse, which is known to be an unusually effective way of spreading AIDS because it involves depositing semen, a fluid carrying the virus, inside the body of another person. Not all homosexuals, however, engage in anal intercourse; many homosexuals never practice anal intercourse. On the other hand, an unknown number of heterosexuals do. So, it is anal inter-course—not sexual orientation—that presents the risk of infection.

It is not known exactly how widespread anal intercourse is in our society, but it is well established that heterosexuals have en-gaged in anal intercourse as a means of birth control or as a method of sexual enjoyment for centuries. A female partner of an infected heterosexual male is as much at risk from having anal sex with that male partner as a gay man would be. Similarly, a female partner of an infected heterosexual male is as much at risk from having oral sex with that male partner as a gay man would be. It is the *activity* that spreads the virus, not the sexual orientation of the people engaging in the activity.

The distinction becomes critical in cases where individuals en-gage in specific risk activities but do not self-identify with the label of a risk group and therefore do not appreciate the risk being taken. The example of a woman being at risk when having unprotected anal intercourse with a man is fairly obvious. They are certainly not engaging in homosexual activity, but she is definitely at risk if he is a carrier. Less obvious but more common is the case of a "heterosexual male" having unprotected anal intercourse or some other form of sexual activity with another "heterosexual male," both viewing themselves as "straight" and therefore not at risk for AIDS. Labels, particularly labels involving "belonging" to a "risk group" for AIDS, are too often a matter of subjective self-identity, and can be dangerously misleading. If the insertive sex partner is carrying the AIDS virus in his semen, anal intercourse without a condom is extremely risky for the receptive partner, regardless of the receptive partner's gender, and regardless of his or her self-perceived sexual orientation.

Conversely, when two women engage in sex with one another they are engaging in homosexual activity, but they are at a low risk for AIDS. The activities in which they are engaged generally do not carry substantial risk. Sexual orientation is not the issue. The specific sexual activities and the specific opportunities to move the virus from inside one body to inside another body are what matter. Female-to-female sexual encounters rarely transmit venereal disease. Lesbians can get AIDS, but generally it is through sex with men or by sharing IV drug needles, not because of anything specifically having to do with being lesbian.

Oral Sex and AIDS Risk   Anal intercourse is well documented as an effective means of spreading the AIDS virus. The situation with oral sex is far less certain. The risk assessment of oral transmission of the AIDS virus has a theoretical basis only. If semen or vaginal fluids carry the virus, and if these fluids enter the mouth and digestive system of the sexual partner, and if the virus were then to find an entry point within the mouth, gums or digestive system, infection could occur. But the virus could not enter those tissues if the tissues were intact, which would ordinarily be the case. Only if there were lesions or ulcers, or perhaps periodontal disease of the gums, could the virus find a way into the bloodstream. The mouth and digestive system are remarkably well defended against bacteria and other disease-causing agents. The enzymes of the mouth and the digestive acids of the stomach would very likely kill the virus. Nevertheless, the theoretical risk of oral transmission of the AIDS virus exists and needs to be considered.

Oral sex with a man to climax is a considerably greater risk since the AIDS virus could be present in a fairly large quantity. Oral sex with a woman would be at lower risk since the quantity of infected vaginal fluid ingested would be less.

Two large studies of the AIDS-related sexual risks of homosexual men, one in San Francisco, co-sponsored by the University of

California and Children's Hospital, and another conducted independently in Canada, compared the sexual histories of gay men to their AIDS antibody status and actual diagnoses of AIDS. In both studies, computer correlations between AIDS status and sexual history indicated that the men who engaged only in oral sex were only a little more likely to be infected with AIDS than those who had been celibate or had engaged only in practices such as masturbation. In other words, neither study could find much risk in oral sex based on actual case histories.

Under the American system of health care, our federal government is responsible for providing research about the way diseases are spread. Our federal government barely recognizes the existence of vaginal sex, let alone oral sex. It is unlikely that federal research projects will ever specifically investigate the safety of oral sex, even for heterosexuals. Many people tend to forget that oral sex between heterosexuals is still illegal in a number of states. Federal policy has been such that if an activity is illegal anywhere in the country, the government will not advise its citizens on the safe performance of the illegal activity. It is unlikely that the issue of the safety of oral sex will be resolved soon, but for now, all that can be said is that the risk is fairly low.

Vaginal Sex and AIDS Risk   A few years ago a debate raged as to whether heterosexuals could transmit AIDS through vaginal sex. The debate is now settled: AIDS transmission can definitely occur during vaginal sex, either from men to women or from women to men. The risks, however, are not equal between male and female partners. The risk of AIDS transmission during vaginal sex is substantially higher for the female partner than for the male partner. If the male partner is a carrier of the virus, at ejaculation a large quantity of virus-laden semen is deposited inside the woman's body, and finds its way through mucous membranes into the woman's bloodstream. As is the case with anal sex, the receptive partner is at far greater risk than the insertive partner.

The male partner is at a lower risk: If the female partner's vaginal secretions contain virus-laden lymphocytes, the virus could enter through any cut or sore on the penis, or the vaginal secretions could be forced up the urethra and find an entry through its mucous membranes. For obvious reasons, women are less "efficient" sexual transmitters of the AIDS virus than men, but males have contracted AIDS from vaginal sex with infected women. Again, a condom, properly used, can prevent transmission.

Knowing Who Is Infected with the Virus   It is impossible to tell if a person has AIDS by looking at him or her. It is not really possible to know whether a person is carrying the virus or not. A person can acquire the virus from one method and pass it on through another. For example, a bisexual male could acquire the virus by having anal sex with an infected male. This newly infected male could then pass on the virus to a heterosexual female through sex. The woman could then pass it on by sharing a needle with another person regardless of that person's gender or sexual orientation. The fourth person could then pass on the virus to someone else, male or female, through any of the other methods. An infected female who becomes pregnant could infect her unborn child.

You cannot tell by looking at a person if he or she is carrying the AIDS virus. Not even experienced AIDS medical specialists can tell by looking. You cannot tell by asking, since there is no guarantee that the person will tell the truth, nor is there any guarantee that the person will know his or her HIV status. Nor can one accurately assess by looking at or talking with someone, or even by knowing someone for many years, whether that person engages in bisexual activity or uses IV drugs, or could otherwise have been exposed to the virus through a blood-contact method.

For many people, their sexual activities are among the most private aspects of their life. Drug use is often concealed even from close friends. Married people can be unaware of their spouse's infidelities even after years of marriage. Few beliefs about AIDS and sex are so foolish or so deadly as the belief that "I can tell who has it and who doesn't." You cannot. The only safe procedure when having sex with a new partner is to behave as if one or both of you may be a carrier, and use a condom—always.

The Search for a Vaccine

It is still too early to predict with any certainty at what point a vaccine or cure for AIDS would be available. Research efforts on both are underway. It is important to remember, though, that medical research is an agonizingly slow process. Spectacular medical breakthroughs sometimes occur, but they occur more commonly in science fiction than in the course of everyday scientific research.

Whenever the press reports that a scientist has made a "breakthrough" in AIDS research, it is almost always a breakthrough only in the eyes of other scientists. At this stage in AIDS research, a breakthrough is more accurately an "advance"—that is, an important step leading to other important steps that might someday bring about the desired end result. There have been dozens of "breakthroughs" in AIDS research announced in the press over the past few years, yet in practical terms, we are no closer to an effective vaccine.

There is ample evidence at this point to suggest two significant notions about the future of AIDS as a disease:

1. While it is theoretically possible to develop and produce a preventive AIDS vaccine for distribution to the public, it would be optimistic to expect that a reliable vaccine for AIDS would be ready for general use before the mid-1990s. Vaccines take time to develop, test and produce in quantity. It took decades to develop a vaccine for polio. The more recent development of a vaccine for hepatitis B, a far easier task than developing an

AIDS vaccine, took nearly as long. No one has ever produced a vaccine for a retrovirus, the special class of virus involved in AIDS. Genetic engineering techniques will speed up the development process for the AIDS vaccine, but these experimental new techniques still require time.

Even if an AIDS vaccine were developed in a research lab, several years of testing would be required before it could be widely distributed. The unusually long incubation period for this disease dictates an unusually long trial period. Vaccine trials in humans are risky, and many complex legal and products' liability issues have to be dealt with in significantly new ways before any drug manufacturer would risk exposing large segments of the population to a vaccine that held the potential of *giving* AIDS to some percentage of the population rather than protecting against it.

When a newly developed vaccine is proved to be both safe and effective, more time will be needed just to get manufacturing capacity to the point where enough vaccine could be produced for the tens of millions of Americans who eagerly seek immunity to AIDS. That projection doesn't even consider the inevitable strong demand for the vaccine in every major country outside the U.S., or the far greater need for mass inoculation of hundreds of millions of people in Third World countries. A more realistic target for a tested, approved, mass-produced and marketable vaccine for AIDS would be near the *end* of the 1990s.

2. It is also theoretically possible to develop a cure for AIDS; however, it is not likely to occur in this century. What we are far more likely to see is the development of a maintenance drug that would "freeze" the virus in status quo, preventing it from reproducing and blocking it from infecting any additional lymphocytes. So long as such a drug regimen were continued, the patient could remain in at least a status quo condition without

getting worse. If administered early enough in the infection process, the patient could remain healthy so long as the drug was continued, and so long as the drug itself had no serious side-effects.

A maintenance drug for people carrying the AIDS virus would be analogous to the daily insulin requirement of diabetics. So long as the proper dose of insulin is administered on a regular basis, diabetics can generally lead normal lives. Their health is dependent, though, on a continuing resupply of the drug. The most probable scenario, then, for AIDS patients and virus carriers would be a daily drug regimen—for the rest of their lives—that would prevent the virus from causing further damage to the body's lymphocytes, until such time as a cure was available.

Understanding the Role of Antibodies

Antibodies are protein substances manufactured by the human immune system to help defend us against diseases. The body makes a specific antibody for each disease we encounter. If we are exposed to a measles virus, the immune system will develop antibodies specifically designed to attack measles viruses. If we are exposed to chickenpox, our bodies will produce an antibody that will attach itself only to a chickenpox virus. A very specific antibody will be produced by the immune system for each disease to which we have been exposed.

These antibodies are produced by the B cells in our lymph glands. Lymph glands become swollen during an infection, because the body is busy making antibodies in those glands; the glands swell in order to increase production of the necessary antibodies. Swollen lymph glands, then, are evidence that the body is busy manufacturing antibodies to some outside invader.

A great deal has been learned recently about the immune mechanisms of our bodies, including the role of antibodies. The human immune system is an amazing interplay of microscopic particles, each one of which plays a highly specialized role in a complex but remarkably well coordinated system that allows us to lead remarkably healthy lives most of the time. When you consider that our bodies are under constant attack by all sorts of organisms twenty-four hours every day, and when you consider how rarely we are ill, the effectiveness of our immune response becomes apparent.

The purpose of each different type of antibody developed by the immune system is to attach itself to an invading disease particle, and to identify that attacker by a chemical signal or flag. The chemical signal can be recognized by other defensive organisms in our bodies. One of the immune system's defensive components, for example, is a cell called a macrophage. The word macrophage means "big eater." Macrophages are something like a cross between a Pac Man and a vacuum cleaner. It's their job to remove viruses and bacteria that don't belong in our bodies. These macrophages respond to chemical signals produced by the antibodies that in effect say to the macrophage, "come eat me and whatever I'm attached to." The antibody serves as a "flag" to identify something that doesn't belong in our bodies so that other defensive cells in our immune system—like the macrophages—can take appropriate action to get rid of the offending invader.

Once the body has identified a specific invader and has prepared antibodies specifically for that invader, the antibodies tend to remain in our bodies for life. So, if we had measles and chickenpox as children, we will have antibodies to measles and chickenpox in our blood for the rest of our lives. Should we ever be exposed to measles or chickenpox again, the specific antibodies would instantly respond, and the invader would be eliminated before it could gain a foothold. Thus we say that we have an "immunity" to measles and chickenpox. We can't get those diseases again—or more accurately, those diseases can't get us again—because our bodies are prepared in advance and will knock out those diseases from the first moment of exposure.

Vaccines Trigger Production of Antibodies

We have all taken vaccines—we have "been vaccinated," we say—against several diseases: diphtheria, smallpox, polio, for example. We take them on faith but we don't really understand how vaccines operate within our bodies.

The purpose of a vaccine is to "trick" the body into thinking that it has been invaded by a specific disease so that the B cells in the body will manufacture antibodies to that specific disease. So, a polio vaccine tricks our body into making antibodies to the polio virus. The antibodies will then float around our bloodstream in readiness for years, just waiting for the real disease to come along. If we are later exposed to that disease for which we've been vaccinated, the antibodies are waiting like a protective army to quickly eliminate the invader. A vaccine against, say, polio, means that the body's defenses are already prepared against polio. The vaccine is often made from dead or weakened disease organisms that trigger the body's mechanism without being strong enough to actually cause the disease.

The presence of AIDS antibodies in the bloodstream—which can be detected by a simple blood test—indicates whether or not the AIDS virus was ever present in our body long enough to cause the production of antibodies to it. A positive result on an AIDS antibody test is strong evidence that the virus is probably still present in the body.

Antibody Testing

Because AIDS is such a hidden disease due to its long incubation period, the antibody test can be an important one for anyone who might have reason to be concerned about past exposure. It is not an ideal test, but it is the best one currently available. At some point, a test will be developed that measures the presence of the virus itself—a far more important measure than the presence of antibodies. Until such a virus (or "antigen") test is available, the antibody test is the only way of knowing whether one has been infected with the AIDS virus, without having to wait for years until clinical symptoms of AIDS finally develop. The antibody test is the best early warning device available.

The AIDS antibody test is available almost everywhere in America. Many health departments provide the test at no charge, or at minimum charge. Many health departments also provide extensive information about AIDS and about the test, and provide counseling for those needing it. We strongly advise anyone considering the test to use the counseling services available.

In some states, the test is offered anonymously without any identification being taken; in other jurisdictions, a positive test is reported to health authorities, but under conditions of confidentiality. Many private doctors offer the test, although the patient should first inquire whether the result will become part of the medical record and therefore accessible to insurance companies. Interested persons should call their local health department for information. Be sure to find out the ground rules concerning who has access to your test results. Serious discrimination can result from misuse of the information.

The AIDS antibody test is about as accurate as most other blood tests. However, there are two specific limitations you should know about.

First, there are different brands of antibody tests made by different manufacturers. Different brands of tests have different strengths and weaknesses. You will probably not know what brand of test you are being given. The most popular test—called ELISA—tends to produce excessive false positives, so many health departments confirm all ELISA positives with another, more expensive test— the Western Blot—to eliminate the risk of inaccurate positives. Not all labs follow this important confirming procedure, however, and there will be some percentage of people who are told they have been infected with the virus when in fact they have not.

Second, the body does not produce antibodies immediately upon exposure. Production of antibodies takes from six weeks to six months or longer. During that interim, the infected person would not yet have enough antibodies for the test to register. These persons would test negative when they are in fact infected. A second test six months later is advisable if exposure could have taken place within a short time of the original test.

Therefore, like any other test, the AIDS antibody test is capable of both false positives and false negatives. Given the seriousness of the consequences of inaccurate information from this test, serious misjudgments or discriminations could be made on the basis of false and misleading information. For this reason, mass nonvoluntary testing is definitely counterproductive. Mass education, not mass testing, is still the most effective means of solving this epidemic.

"Antibody Negative" Identification Cards   Some commercial organizations, and a few sex-related clubs, have taken up the practice of issuing "Negative ID cards" to people who have tested negative on the antibody test. The theory—a very dangerous and irresponsible theory—is that such people don't need to practice safe sex.

Negative ID cards are worth no more than the paper they are printed on, and are valid, at best, for the length of time it takes the ink to dry. The Negative card is no guarantee that the person is really negative, even when the test was given, and certainly no guarantee that the person hasn't since been infected. Anyone who would risk their life based on someone's presentation of one of these worthless cards needs to take an IQ test, in addition to an antibody test.

AIDS Prevention Is Not Complicated

AIDS prevention requires only diligence and common sense. Vaginal sex, like anal sex, can transmit the virus. Heterosexual sex, like homosexual sex, can transmit the virus. You cannot tell by looking or talking with someone whether they are a carrier. You cannot depend on an ID card. Condoms can prevent contact with infected semen or vaginal secretions, and should be the keystone of safe sex practices.

Sex partners rarely communicate well about issues like safe sex and condoms. Communication, however, is critical when lives are at stake. It may be awkward and embarrassing to bring up the issue of condoms and AIDS with a new sex partner, but you'll survive your embarrassment. You'll get over the blushed face, the awkward moment. You won't so easily get over AIDS, or the ultimate knowledge that you had transmitted this disease to someone else.

AIDS prevention needs to become routine for the duration of this epidemic. Condom use needs to become so routine that they don't even need to be argued about. In the meantime, lives are at stake, and you can make a difference. Your simple courage and common sense can stop an epidemic. Rarely are ordinary people given such responsibility for the lives of others. We are all fully capable of managing that responsibility. We are all fully capable of stopping the spread of AIDS.

7 ‖ The Future of Corporate Responsibility and Employee Health

This is the first major fatal epidemic since the development of professional and scientific management within the business community. The opportunity exists within the workplace environment to see that AIDS is managed responsibly, rationally, with full recognition of the scientific facts and with some degree of compassion and forethought. Employers have the clearest and most direct channels of communication to enormous numbers of people. Employers have the credibility to effectively communicate and objectively handle emotional and controversial subjects, and they have the financial motivation to take advantage of opportunities for disease prevention. Employers will pay much of the cost of this epidemic. The business community has so far provided most of the demonstrated leadership for sensible approaches to the management of the AIDS epidemic, and that potential has been barely tapped.

AIDS Will Be an Ongoing Issue for the Next Decade

While the AIDS epidemic has not spread "like wildfire" as some early alarmists projected, it has nevertheless spread across certain segments of society that engage in the sexual and drug-using activities that allow the disease to be spread from person to person. In our culture, millions of people have sex with millions of people. At a minimum, tens of thousands of Americans daily share drug needles.

The most recent targets for growing numbers of AIDS infections are urban minority groups—Blacks and Hispanics—and teenagers of all races. The degree to which adolescents experiment with sex and drugs provides a frightening potential for increased AIDS infections. The degree to which the AIDS virus will penetrate into these two populations is not yet clear; it is clear, however, that, because of the topics involved, sex and drugs, government at all levels will be very reluctant to provide the necessary preventive information. In fact, government has been generally paralyzed since the beginning of the AIDS epidemic because of the overwhelming sensitivity of the political issues raised.

As a consequence of the lack of organized prevention programs, because of the very nature of the way AIDS is spread, and as a result of the big head start the virus already has in our society, the AIDS epidemic can be expected to continue throughout the decade of the 1990s. The large number of people already infected and silently incubating the disease guarantees tens of thousands of new cases for the next several years. In planning for organizational approaches to AIDS in the workplace, it is important to bear in mind that this is a long-term issue.

The way to face the AIDS epidemic is to *face* the AIDS epidemic. There are no shortcuts to informing our citizens about this disease, no easy shortcuts to, or convenient substitutes for, responsible individual behavior, or responsible corporate behavior. And there is no better place in which to educate and inform masses of people about this disease than in the workplace.

AIDS would be a fairly straightforward, even simple, public health management matter if there were not such strongly held, often highly emotional, points of view about the relationship of morality and religion to the AIDS epidemic, and strongly held points of view as to what ought to be done about that relationship.

There are still those who argue that AIDS is the result of sin. There are those on the other side who argue that AIDS results from society's stubborn unwillingness to be realistic and honest about sexuality and drug use. For management, these are no-win controversies.

Management's task is to responsibly manage its operating environment and the important relationship with its employees in a way that is rational and predictable, that promotes employee cooperation and loyalty, that complies with the law, and that respects the ultimate bottom-line profitability of the business. Morality, a changing concept at best, and one on which there are divergent and emotional views, is an issue about which one person's opinion may be just as valid as that of another person. There is certainly no objective way to compute or scientifically analyze a resolution of the disagreements.

The juxtaposition of human sexuality, morality and religion generates highly emotional controversies that are unresolvable by any conventional method of analysis or logic. For business and other employers, management of AIDS in the workplace will require steering a cautious course, one that (1) promotes the free and full dissemination of information about AIDS to everyone who needs it; that (2) treats people with AIDS under the label "our employees, our responsibility"; that (3) complies with federal and state laws, including those preventing discrimination against the handicapped, as well as laws and traditions protecting employee confidentiality; and that (4) simultaneously keeps the organization out of the emotional and hopelessly unresolvable debates about morality and religion. There is no fundamental reason why responsible and objective management, acting with integrity, courage and clarity of purpose, would not prove equal to this challenge.

Success Stories Abound

Earlier we mentioned New England Telephone's employee walk-out in May 1985, conducted in front of the local television news cameras, all because there was a person with AIDS working in the facility. It's only fair to mention that the story had a happy ending. Both the initial crisis and the happy ending are typical of corporate experiences about AIDS on the job.

According to Anthony Sprauve of the phone company's parent, NYNEX, shortly after the walkout incident in Boston, a task force of senior managers from the Human Resources, Labor Relations, Legal and Medical departments drafted a company policy on AIDS, which was unanimously approved by the officers of the company. Their AIDS-specific policy is a model of brevity:

> New England Telephone's position is that AIDS is treated like any other illness contracted by an employee.
>
> Accordingly, if an employee is diagnosed as having AIDS, but isn't disabled from working, the employee can return to work. If an employee with AIDS has work limitations, the Company will make reasonable accommodations.

On the evening of the walkout, the company, in conjunction with the union, conducted an educational meeting for employees and their families. The co-workers returned to work the next day. The AIDS-affected employee's return to work thereafter proceeded smoothly.

New England Telephone decided to undertake what they describe as "one of the most aggressive and pro-active employee education programs on AIDS of any company in the Northeast." The first phase of the program began in June 1987, when the company mailed a brochure explaining the latest medical facts about AIDS to each employee's home. The brochure was accompanied by a letter from the company's medical director that clearly explained New England Telephone's policy on AIDS in the workplace.

While the company "continues to evaluate and assess its efforts to give employees the latest information on this disease," Sprauve also fairly points out that the Boston-based company had to learn "how to handle this subject before the benefits of pro-active AIDS education in the workplace became apparent to the business world at large." Their experience with the issue since instituting mass education programs has been generally positive, and no further incidents of the type described have occurred.

The New England Telephone experience is typical: Without education, AIDS is a serious problem; with education, AIDS is very manageable. Most organizations have been very pleased with the practical results of their programs, and with the typically very positive employee responses.

Case Management of Costs

A public utility company in the Southeast reported that its first eight AIDS cases totaled nearly $1 million in medical expenses. On the other hand, the Bank of America reports that the cost of its cases of AIDS averaged only $25,000 per employee from diagnosis to death. The press reports that in New York, the typical case of AIDS may cost $100,000 in medical expenses; in San Francisco, by contrast, the typical medical bill for an AIDS patient is about $35,000. Why these dramatic differences? The differences are due mostly to "case management" of costs and the extensive use of outpatient and nontraditional resources.

Some employer health organizations—the Washington Business Group on Health is a pioneering example—have argued for some time that case management is necessary in order to get any control over medical costs, particularly for catastrophic illnesses. Case management allows the company's benefits people to do what makes sense in a given case, rather than being restricted to formulas and other kinds of limitations. Case management allows for greater flexibility over the employee's medical treatment. Case management allows greater use of outpatient facilities, home care and home nursing and alternative therapies, all of which in many cases provide far better treatment for the patient at dramatically lower cost for the employer. Case management benefits both the ill employee and the employer.

Ron Colby, Vice President of Group Underwriting and Actuarial Services for Lincoln National Life Insurance Company in Fort Wayne, Indiana, advises that "by 1991, at least two to five percent of all group health claims will be for AIDS, ARC or related conditions. The most immediate and obvious impact on group medical plans will be an increased cost to employers to provide those plans. AIDS will impact benefits costs for all businesses, regardless of their size or location."

Benefits plans, he suggests, should treat AIDS identically to other major illnesses, such as heart disease or cancer. "Case management will necessarily grow in importance. Case management is the efficient coordination of resources for catastrophic illnesses or injuries, usually through the intervention of an experienced case management nurse. The primary focus is on quality alternative care at the lowest possible cost, utilizing services such as home health care and hospice care." Colby concludes that there is significant potential for reducing the average cost of an AIDS claim through case management, and advises that "case management will likely emerge as a key strategy to deliver care-effective and cost-effective medical services to AIDS patients."

The experience of companies using case management for major illnesses confirms his view. A failure to plan for case management, not only for AIDS, but for cancer and other major illnesses, exposes an employer to horrendous medical costs, without providing even the best care for the ill patient. AIDS is serving as a useful motivation for many employers to investigate the advantages of case management as a feature of their medical benefits programs. The overall result will be more effective management of medical costs.

Inter-Company Cooperation and AIDS

"The AIDS epidemic is prompting an unusual degree of cooperation and sharing of information and educational resources among private sector groups," reports health policy analyst Pat Franks, who coordinates a national AIDS resource program for the huge

New Jersey-based Robert Wood Johnson Foundation. Companies are pooling resources to establish AIDS in the workplace policies, and to prepare educational materials.

The Business Leadership Task Force of the Bay Area was an organization of the CEOs of the San Francisco area's largest companies. In 1985, the Business Leadership Task Force set up a working group from seven of the companies to commission the preparation of AIDS in the workplace educational materials, including a video- tape, and to organize a major educational forum about AIDS for local corporate executives. This joint effort by a multi-company committee produced some of the best materials on the subject yet produced.

In New Orleans, Southeast Louisiana Health Cost Management, a business coalition serving the greater New Orleans area and focused on corporate health issues, joined with the Metropolitan Hospital Council of New Orleans and the Orleans Parish Medical Society in January 1986 to conduct a significant seminar for the business world about AIDS. According to its Executive Director, Linda Lambert, the organization's Medicine/Industry Task Force, composed of four representatives from business and four presidents of area medical societies, prepared a policy development guide entitled "Points for Consideration in Developing Policy for Assisting Employees with Life Threatening Illnesses." SLHCM's work is an excellent example of public agency and business organization cooperation.

In October 1987, Allstate Insurance Company sponsored a national corporate conference on AIDS. The result of the conference was a pooling of the participants' creative expertise and the development of the manual "AIDS: Corporate America Responds." The manual addresses the broad spectrum of concerns about AIDS ranging from human resources to corporate philanthropy.

Experiences to date suggest strongly that major employers should join with other local or industry organizations to prepare consistent, multi-organization approaches to AIDS policy and educational issues. Since the fundamental issues are the same for virtually all employers, a multi-employer approach is often better received by employees, and may more easily serve as a role model for smaller organizations.

Managing the Community Environment

The attitudes about AIDS within an employee group cannot be wholly divorced from general attitudes about AIDS within society, no matter how much education you do for employees at work. Unfortunately, but inevitably, the political arena has much to do with how the public—and your employees and their families—will view this very politicized disease. Managing AIDS in the workplace also requires using your organizational influence within your community to assure rational public policies about AIDS: policies that fit the scientific facts, policies that are based on considerations of public health, policies that focus on solving the medical and public health problems associated with this disease, policies that are free of hysteria and other agendas.

Public calls for quarantine of AIDS-infected people, for firing AIDS-infected people from certain kinds of jobs, for mandating AIDS antibody testing, are politically motivated proposals having nothing really to do with ending or controlling the AIDS epidemic. Nevertheless, these proposals—based as they are on the notion of casual transmission of AIDS—stir up public fears and paranoia about this disease. In most cases, such proposals are expressly designed to do so in order to further other agendas having nothing to do with AIDS at all. AIDS is simply being used as a convenient excuse for some long-standing social goals of certain political groups. AIDS phobia unfortunately still plays well in the press, as any review of the covers of the *National Enquirer* and other publications at the supermarket checkout will demonstrate. AIDS phobia also plays well with certain political groups.

Employers have a vested interest in minimizing the impact of such irresponsible proposals, as well as a vested interest in maximiz-

ing sensible public policies about AIDS. The public is easily confused by the kind of propositions that suggest AIDS is casually
spread. That kind of confusion and uncertainty makes more
difficult the management of AIDS-related issues on the job. Employers have a responsibility—to themselves and to their employees—to promote sane public policy approaches to the AIDS
epidemic, and to oppose political measures based principally on
hysteria and fear.

Medical ethicist Nora K. Bell, Ph.D., Chair of the Department
of Philosophy at the University of South Carolina, reminds us that

> those who urge that we have a duty to society to control and eradicate
> this horrible disease sometimes also urge that individual rights have to
> be compromised in the effort. They portray the moral dilemma in com-
> batting AIDS as requiring that we choose whether to affirm individual
> rights or the good of society. Because AIDS is so difficult to spread,
> virtually no social or health care context requires a choice between
> whether to protect the individual or to protect society.
>
> Rather, controlling the spread of AIDS means enacting laws to deter
> discrimination; it means enforcing confidentiality with strict sanctions
> and fines, allowing exceptions only in those contexts where spread is
> known to be likely. There is no medical or scientific justification for
> policies that would isolate or quarantine or publicly identify the infected.
>
> Controlling the spread of AIDS means coming to terms with the fact
> that compassion and control are not mutually exclusive. Controlling the
> spread of AIDS means acknowledging that there is no medical warrant
> for compromising individual rights in fighting this disease. In attempting
> to combat AIDS, we are not on the horns of a dilemma. One can continue
> to affirm both individual rights and the good of society.

Public policies based on fear, distrust of medical information,
hysteria or superstition, or which treat certain segments of society
as "disposable" in the interest of protecting "normal people," or
which institutionalize and legitimatize paranoia or bias, make more
difficult the management job to be accomplished in the workplace.

Corporate influence should not ignore these important aspects of the public response to AIDS because of the impact that such public policy measures have among employees on the job.

Corporate Responsibility, Corporate Opportunity

Whether we like it or not, AIDS is a part of our generation's world. Our generation has the opportunity—and indeed the responsibility—to respond to this deadly epidemic with intelligent and rational reactions. Hysteria and paranoia only compound a terrible situation in which thousands of our fellow citizens have died, and in which hundreds of thousands will undoubtedly die over time if—as seems to be the case—science is unable to unlock the mysteries of an AIDS cure in time.

AIDS is a slow, disfiguring, crippling illness, leading sadly down a spiral path to death. Those who contract it need our support. We have a responsibility to our fellow humans not to abandon or discard them when they most need our care and our concern. Employees who contract AIDS have the right to assume that their employer will fulfill its contract to provide medical care and disability benefits, will give them a chance for reasonable accommodation, and will continue to regard these employees as part of its work family. Any other approach is tragic, and will not serve to the credit of our generation of managers. We are capable of better. History will judge the integrity of our response.

If other employees initially find difficult the acceptance of an AIDS patient within their midst, managers have two simple choices: (1) We can allow our companies to be ruled by irrational fears, and by a wholesale disregard of fact and logic and reasonableness, and hope that we have not thereby set a pattern for other issues in the future; or (2) we can provide information and education for co-workers, and base our employment decisions on scientific proof, logic and simple human decency.

The policy among the pioneering organizations who have so far taken a stand about AIDS in the workplace is very clear: *Employees with AIDS are entitled to be treated with the same dignity and concern and support as are employees with any other life-threatening illness.* This policy should serve as a role model for all other organizations.

Our generation of managers, the business community at large, and employers in the government and other nonprofit fields have a unique opportunity to exercise their considerable power to impact the course of the AIDS epidemic in our country. As the Surgeon General and dozens of public health experts have advised repeatedly now for several years, "knowing the facts about AIDS can prevent the spread of the disease. Education of those who risk infecting themselves or infecting other people is the only way we can stop the spread of AIDS." Government legislation is largely incapable of that kind of education.

Employers, not government, have the resources, and the ultimate financial motivation, to provide that education to enormous numbers of people in the workplace. There is no larger "captive audience" to be found in our society, and experience indicates that this audience responds very well to information about this subject when it is presented in the work environment. Employees want the information.

You now have all the necessary facts about AIDS. You have all the information you need to plan your organization's response to AIDS. You have the information you need to begin the process of developing education programs for your employees. All that remains is your commitment to the well-being of your workforce, your commitment to do what obviously needs to be done. How you respond will impact the history of the remainder of this century. The responsibility—and the opportunity—are yours!

Appendix

SURGEON GENERAL'S REPORT ON ACQUIRED IMMUNE DEFICIENCY SYNDROME

U.S. Department of Health and Human Services

Foreword

This is a report from the Surgeon General of the U.S. Public Health Service to the people of the United States on AIDS. Acquired Immune Deficiency Syndrome is an epidemic that has already killed thousands of people, mostly young, productive Americans. In addition to illness, disability, and death, AIDS has brought fear to the hearts of most Americans—fear of disease and fear of the unknown. Initial reporting of AIDS occurred in the United States, but AIDS and the spread of the AIDS virus is an international problem. This report focuses on prevention that could be applied in all countries.

My report will inform you about AIDS, how it is transmitted, the relative risks of infection and how to prevent it. It will help you understand your fears. Fear can be useful when it helps people avoid behavior that puts them at risk for AIDS. On the other hand, unreasonable fear can be as crippling as the disease itself. If you are participating in activities that could expose you to the AIDS virus, this report could save your life.

In preparing this report, I consulted with the best medical and scientific experts this country can offer. I met with leaders of organizations concerned with health, education, and other aspects of our society to gain their views of the problems associated with AIDS. The information in this report is current and timely.

This report was written personally by me to provide the necessary understanding of AIDS.

The vast majority of Americans are against illicit drugs. As a health officer I am opposed to the use of illicit drugs. As a practicing physician for more than forty years, I have seen the devastation that follows the use of illicit drugs—addiction, poor health, family disruption, emotional

153

disturbances and death. I applaud the President's initiative to rid this nation of the curse of illicit drug use and addiction. The success of his initiative is critical to the health of the American people and will also help reduce the number of persons exposed to the AIDS virus.

Some Americans have difficulties in dealing with the subjects of sex, sexual practices, and alternate lifestyles. Many Americans are opposed to homosexuality, promiscuity of any kind, and prostitution. This report must deal with all of these issues, but does so with the intent that information and education can change individual behavior, since this is the primary way to stop the epidemic of AIDS. This report deals with the positive and negative consequences of activities and behaviors from a health and medical point of view.

Adolescents and pre-adolescents are those whose behavior we wish to especially influence because of their vulnerability when they are exploring their own sexuality (heterosexual and homosexual) and perhaps experimenting with drugs. Teenagers often consider themselves immortal, and these young people may be putting themselves at great risk.

Education about AIDS should start in early elementary school and at home so that children can grow up knowing the behavior to avoid to protect themselves from exposure to the AIDS virus. The threat of AIDS can provide an opportunity for parents to instill in their children their own moral and ethical standards.

Those of us who are parents, educators and community leaders, indeed all adults, cannot disregard this responsibility to educate our young. The need is critical and the price of neglect is high. The lives of our young people depend on our fulfilling our responsibility.

AIDS is an infectious disease. It is contagious, but it cannot be spread in the same manner as a common cold or measles or chicken pox. It is contagious in the same way that sexually transmitted diseases, such as syphilis and gonorrhea, are contagious. AIDS can also be spread through the sharing of intravenous drug needles and syringes used for injecting illicit drugs.

AIDS is *not* spread by common everyday contact but by sexual contact (penis-vagina, penis-rectum, mouth-rectum, mouth-vagina, mouth-penis). Yet there is great misunderstanding resulting in unfounded fear that AIDS can be spread by casual, non-sexual contact. The first cases of AIDS were reported in this country in 1981. We would know by now if AIDS were passed by casual, non-sexual contact.

Today those practicing high risk behavior who become infected with the AIDS virus are found mainly among homosexual and bisexual men and male and female intravenous drug users. Heterosexual transmission is expected to account for an increasing proportion of those who become infected with the AIDS virus in the future.

At the beginning of the AIDS epidemic many Americans had little sympathy for people with AIDS. The feeling was that somehow people from certain groups "deserved" their illness. Let us put those feelings behind us. We are fighting a disease, not people. Those who are already afflicted are sick people and need our care as do all sick patients. The country must face this epidemic as a unified society. We must prevent the spread of AIDS while at the same time preserving our humanity and intimacy.

AIDS is a life-threatening disease and a major public health issue. Its impact on our society is and will continue to be devastating. By the end of 1991, an estimated 270,000 cases of AIDS will have occurred with 179,000 deaths within the decade since the disease was first recognized. In the year 1991, an estimated 145,000 patients with AIDS will need health and supportive services at a total cost of between $8 and $16 billion. However, AIDS is preventable. It can be controlled by changes in personal behavior. It is the responsibility of every citizen to be informed about AIDS and to exercise the appropriate preventive measures. This report will tell you how.

The spread of AIDS can and must be stopped.

C. Everett Koop, M.D., ScD.
Surgeon General

AIDS

AIDS Caused by Virus   The letters A-I-D-S stand for Acquired
Immune Deficiency Syndrome. When a person is sick with AIDS, he/she
is in the final stages of a series of health problems caused by a virus
(germ) that can be passed from one person to another chiefly during
sexual contact or through the sharing of intravenous drug needles and
syringes used for "shooting" drugs. Scientists have named the AIDS
virus "HIV or HTLV-III or LAV"[1]. These abbreviations stand for information denoting a virus that attacks white blood cells (T-Lymphocytes)
in the human blood. Throughout this publication, we will call the virus
the "AIDS virus." The AIDS virus attacks a person's immune system
and damages his/her ability to fight other disease. Without a functioning
immune system to ward off other germs, he/she now becomes vulnerable
to becoming infected by bacteria, protozoa, fungi, and other viruses and

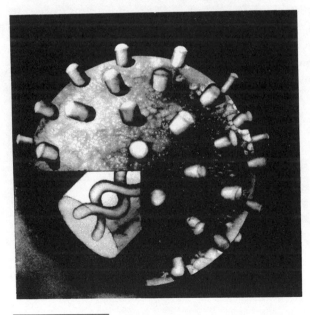

*Artist's drawing of
AIDS virus with cut-
away view showing
genetic (reproductive)
material.*

[1]These are different names given to AIDS virus by the scientific community:

HIV   –Human Immunodeficiency Virus
HTLV-III–Human T-Lymphotropic Virus Type III
LAV   –Lymphadenopathy Associated Virus

malignancies, which may cause life-threatening illness, such as pneumonia, meningitis, and cancer.

No Known Cure   There is presently no cure for AIDS. There is presently no vaccine to prevent AIDS.

Virus Invades Blood Stream   When the AIDS virus enters the blood stream, it begins to attack certain white blood cells (T-Lymphocytes). Substances called antibodies are produced by the body. These antibodies can be detected in the blood by a simple test, usually two weeks to three months after infection. Even before the antibody test is positive, the victim can pass the virus to others by methods that will be explained.

Once an individual is infected, there are several possibilities. Some people may remain well but even so they are able to infect others. Others may develop a disease that is less serious than AIDS referred to as AIDS-Related Complex (ARC). In some people the protective immune system may be destroyed by the virus and then other germs (bacteria, protozoa, fungi and other viruses) and cancers that ordinarily would never get a foothold cause "opportunistic diseases"—using the *opportunity* of lowered resistance to infect and destroy. Some of the most common are *Pneumocystis carinii* pneumonia and tuberculosis. Individuals infected with the AIDS virus may also develop certain types of cancers such as Kaposi's sarcoma. These infected people have classic AIDS. Evidence shows that the AIDS virus may also attack the nervous system, causing damage to the brain.

Signs and Symptoms

No Signs   Some people remain apparently well after infection with the AIDS virus. They may have no physically apparent symptoms of illness. However, if proper precautions are not used with sexual contacts and/or intravenous drug use, these infected individuals can spread the virus to others. Anyone who thinks he or she is infected or involved in high risk behaviors should not donate his/her blood, organs, tissues, or sperm because they may now contain the AIDS virus.

ARC   AIDS-Related Complex (ARC) is a condition caused by the AIDS virus in which the patient tests positive for AIDS infection and has a specific set of clinical symptoms. However, ARC patients' symptoms are often less severe than those with the disease we call classic AIDS. Signs and symptoms of ARC may include loss of appetite, weight loss, fever, night sweats, skin rashes, diarrhea, tiredness, lack of resistance to infection, or swollen lymph nodes. These are also signs and symptoms of many other diseases and a physician should be consulted.

AIDS   Only a qualified health professional can diagnose AIDS, which is the result of a natural progress of infection by the AIDS virus. AIDS destroys the body's immune (defense) system and allows otherwise controllable infections to invade the body and cause additional diseases. These opportunistic diseases would not otherwise gain a foothold in the body. These opportunistic diseases may eventually cause death.

Some symptoms and signs of AIDS and the "opportunistic infections" may include a persistent cough and fever associated with shortness of breath or difficult breathing and may be the symptoms of *Pneumocystis carinii* pneumonia. Multiple purplish blotches and bumps on the skin may be a sign of Kaposi's sarcoma. The AIDS virus in all infected people is essentially the same; the reactions of individuals may differ.

Long Term   The AIDS virus may also attack the nervous system and cause delayed damage to the brain. This damage may take years to develop and the symptoms may show up as memory loss, indifference, loss of coordination, partial paralysis, or mental disorder. These symptoms may occur alone, or with other symptoms mentioned earlier.

AIDS: the present situation

The number of people estimated to be infected with the AIDS virus in the United States is about 1.5 million. All of these individuals are assumed to be capable of spreading the virus sexually (heterosexually or homosexually) or by sharing needles and syringes or other implements for intravenous drug use. Of these, an estimated 100,000 to 200,000 will come down with AIDS-Related Complex (ARC). It is difficult to predict the number who will develop ARC or AIDS because symptoms sometimes take as long as nine years to show up. With our present knowledge, scientists predict that 20 to 30 percent of those infected with the AIDS virus will develop an illness that fits an accepted definition of AIDS within five years. The number of persons known to have AIDS in the United States to date is over 25,000; of these, about half have died of the disease. Since there is no cure, the others are expected to also eventually die from their disease.

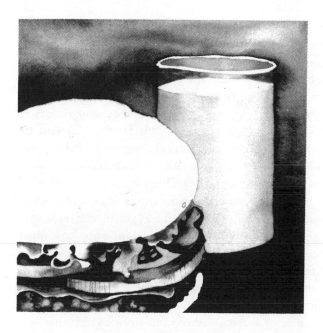

The majority of infected antibody positive individuals who carry the AIDS virus show no disease symptoms and may not come down with the disease for many years, if ever.

No Risk from Casual Contact There is no known risk of non-sexual infection in most of the situations we encounter in our daily lives. We know that family members living with individuals who have the AIDS virus do not become infected except through sexual contact. There is no evidence of transmission (spread) of AIDS virus by everyday contact even though these family members shared food, towels, cups, razors, even toothbrushes, and kissed each other.

Health Workers We know even more about health care workers exposed to AIDS patients. About 2,500 health workers who were caring for AIDS patients when they were sickest have been carefully studied and tested for infection with the AIDS virus. These doctors, nurses and other health care givers have been exposed to the AIDS patients' blood, stool and other body fluids. Approximately 750 of these health workers reported possible additional exposure by direct contact with a patient's body fluid through spills or being accidentally stuck with a needle. Upon testing these 750, only 3 who had accidentally stuck themselves with a needle had a positive antibody test for exposure to the AIDS virus. Because health workers had much more contact with patients and their body fluids than would be expected from common everyday contact, it is clear that the AIDS virus is not transmitted by casual contact.

Control of Certain Behaviors Can Stop Further Spread of AIDS   Knowing the facts about AIDS can prevent the spread of the disease. Education of those who risk infecting themselves or infecting other people is the only way we can stop the spread of AIDS. People must be responsible about their sexual behavior and must avoid the use of illicit intravenous drugs and needle sharing. We will describe the types of behavior that lead to infection by the AIDS virus and the personal measures that must be taken for effective protection. If we are to stop the AIDS epidemic, we all must understand the disease—its cause, its nature, and its prevention. *Precautions must be taken.* The AIDS virus infects persons who expose themselves to known risk behavior, such as certain types of homosexual and heterosexual activities or sharing intravenous drug equipment.

Risks   Although the initial discovery was in the homosexual community, AIDS is not a disease only of homosexuals. AIDS is found in heterosexual people as well. AIDS is not a black or white disease. AIDS is not just a male disease. AIDS is found in women; it is found in children. In the future AIDS will probably increase and spread among people who are not homosexual or intravenous drug abusers in the same manner as other sexually transmitted diseases like syphilis and gonorrhea.

Sex Between Men   Men who have sexual relations with other men are especially at risk. About 70 percent of AIDS victims throughout the country are male homosexuals and bisexuals. This percentage probably will decline as heterosexual transmission increases. *Infection results from a sexual relationship with an infected person.*

Multiple Partners   The risk of infection increases according to the number of sexual partners one has, *male or female.* The more partners you have, the greater the risk of becoming infected with the AIDS virus.

How Exposed   Although the AIDS virus is found in several body fluids, a person acquires the virus during sexual contact with an infected person's blood or semen and possibly vaginal secretions. The virus then enters a person's blood stream through their rectum, vagina or penis.

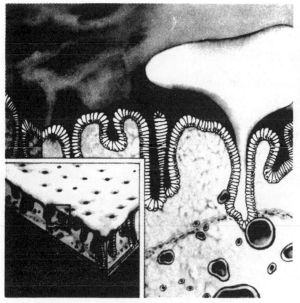

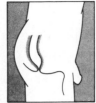

Vulnerable rectum lining provides avenue for entry of AIDS virus into the blood stream.

Small (unseen by the naked eye) tears in the surface lining of the vagina or rectum may occur during insertion of the penis, fingers, or other objects, thus opening an avenue for entrance of the virus directly into the blood stream; therefore, the AIDS virus can be passed from penis to rectum and vagina and vice versa without a visible tear in the tissue or the presence of blood.

Prevention of Sexual Transmission—Know Your Partner

Couples who maintain mutually faithful monogamous relationships (only one continuing sexual partner) are protected from AIDS through sexual transmission. If you have been faithful for at least five years and your partner has been faithful too, neither of you is at risk. If you have not been faithful, then you and your partner are at risk. If your partner has not been faithful, then your partner is at risk which also puts you at risk. This is true for both heterosexual and homosexual couples. Unless it is possible to know with *absolute certainty* that neither you nor your sexual partner is carrying the virus of AIDS, you must use protective behavior. *Absolute certainty* means not only that you and your partner have maintained a mutually faithful monogamous sexual relationship, but it means that neither you nor your partner has used illegal intravenous drugs.

AIDS: you can protect yourself from infection

Some personal measures are adequate to safely protect yourself and others from infection by the AIDS virus and its complications. Among these are:

- If you have been involved in any of the high risk sexual activities described above or have injected illicit intravenous drugs into your body, you should have a blood test to see if you have been infected with the AIDS virus.

- If your test is positive or if you engage in high risk activities and choose not to have a test, you should tell your sexual partner. If you jointly decide to have sex, you must protect your partner by always using a rubber (condom) during (start to finish) sexual intercourse (vagina or rectum).

- If your partner has a positive blood test showing that he/she has been infected with the AIDS virus or you suspect that he/she has been exposed

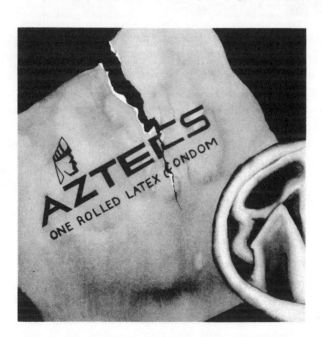

by previous heterosexual or homosexual behavior or use of intravenous drugs with shared needles and syringes, a rubber (condom) during (start to finish) sexual intercourse (vagina or rectum).

- If you or your partner is at high risk, avoid mouth contact with the penis, vagina, or rectum.

- Avoid all sexual activities which could cause cuts or tears in the linings of the rectum, vagina, or penis.

- Single teenage girls have been warned that pregnancy and contracting sexually transmitted diseases can be the result of only one act of sexual intercourse. They have been taught to say *NO* to sex! They have been taught to say *NO* to drugs! By saying *NO* to sex and drugs, they can avoid AIDS which can *kill* them! The same is true for teenage boys who should also not have rectal intercourse with other males. It may result in AIDS.

- Do not have sex with prostitutes. Infected male and female prostitutes are frequently also intravenous drug abusers; therefore, they may infect clients by sexual intercourse and other intravenous drug abusers by sharing their intravenous drug equipment. Female prostitutes also can infect their unborn babies.

Intravenous Drug Users   Drug abusers who inject drugs into their veins are another population group at high risk and with high rates of infection by the AIDS virus. Users of intravenous drugs make up 25 percent of the cases of AIDS throughout the country. The AIDS virus is carried in contaminated blood left in the needle, syringe, or other drug related implements and the virus is injected into the new victim by reusing dirty syringes and needles. Even the smallest amount of infected blood left in a used needle or syringe can contain live AIDS virus to be passed on to the next user of those dirty implements.

No one should shoot up drugs because addiction, poor health, family disruption, emotional disturbances and death could follow. However, many drug users are addicted to drugs and for one reason or another have not changed their behavior. For these people, the only way not to

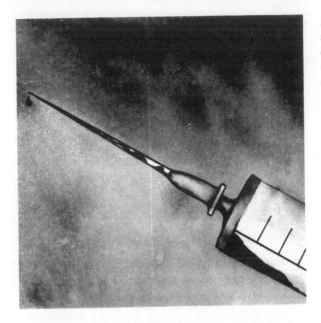

*Dirty intravenous
needle and syringe
contaminated with blood
that may contain the
AIDS virus.*

get AIDS is *to use a clean, previously unused* needle, syringe or any other implement necessary for the injection of the drug solution.

Hemophilia   Some persons with hemophilia (a blood clotting disorder that makes them subject to bleeding) have been infected with the AIDS virus either through blood transfusion or the use of blood products that help their blood clot. Now that we know how to prepare safe blood products to aid clotting, this is unlikely to happen. This group represents a very small percentage of the cases of AIDS throughout the country.

Blood Transfusion   Currently all blood donors are initially screened and blood is *not* accepted from high risk individuals. Blood that has been collected for use is tested for the presence of antibody to the AIDS virus. However, some people may have had a blood transfusion prior to March 1985 before we knew how to screen blood for safe transfusion and may have become infected with the AIDS virus. Fortunately there are not now a large number of these cases. With routine testing of blood products, the blood supply for transfusion is now safer than it has ever been with regard to AIDS.

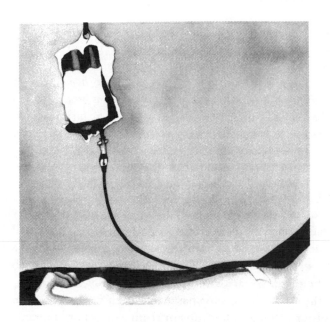

Persons who have engaged in homosexual activities or have shot street drugs within the last 10 years should *never* donate blood.

Mother Can Infect Newborn   If a woman is infected with the AIDS virus and becomes pregnant, she is more likely to develop ARC or classic AIDS, and she can pass the AIDS virus to her unborn child. Approximately one third of the babies born to AIDS-infected mothers will also be infected with the AIDS virus. Most of the infected babies will eventually develop the disease and die. Several of these babies have been born to wives of hemophiliac men infected with the AIDS virus by way of contaminated blood products. Some babies have also been born to women who became infected with the AIDS virus by bisexual partners who had the virus. Almost all babies with AIDS have been born to women who were intravenous drug users or the sexual partners of intravenous drug users who were infected with the AIDS virus. More such babies can be expected.

Think carefully if you plan on becoming pregnant. If there is any chance that you may be in any high risk group or that you have had sex with someone in a high risk group, such as homosexual and bisexual males, drug abusers and their sexual partners, see your doctor.

Summary   *AIDS affects certain groups of the population. Homosexual and bisexual males who have had sexual contact with other homosexual or bisexual males as well as those who "shoot" street drugs are at greatest risk of exposure, infection and eventual death. Sexual partners of these high risk individuals are at risk, as well as any children born to women who carry the virus. Heterosexual persons are increasingly at risk.*

AIDS: what is safe

Most Behavior is Safe   Everyday living does not present any risk of infection. You *cannot* get AIDS from casual social contact. Casual social contact should not be confused with casual *sexual* contact which is a major cause of the spread of the AIDS virus. Casual *social* contact such as shaking hands, hugging, social kissing, crying, coughing or sneezing, will not transmit the AIDS virus. Nor has AIDS been contracted from swimming in pools or bathing in hot tubs or from eating in restaurants (even if a restaurant worker has AIDS or carries the AIDS virus.) AIDS is not contracted from sharing bed linens, towels, cups, straws, dishes, or any other eating utensils. You cannot get AIDS from toilets, doorknobs, telephones, office machinery, or household furniture. You cannot get AIDS from body massages, masturbation or any non-sexual contact.

Donating Blood   Donating blood is *not* risky at all. *You cannot get AIDS by donating blood.*

Receiving Blood   In the U.S. every blood donor is screened to exclude high risk persons and every blood donation is now tested for the presence of antibodies to the AIDS virus. Blood that shows exposure to the AIDS virus by the presence of antibodies is not used either for transfusion or for the manufacture of blood products. Blood banks are as safe as current technology can make them. Because antibodies do not form immediately after exposure to the virus, a newly infected person may unknowingly donate blood after becoming infected but before his/her antibody test becomes positive. It is estimated that this might occur less than once in 100,000 donations.

There is no danger of AIDS virus infection from visiting a doctor, dentist, hospital, hairdresser or beautician. AIDS cannot be transmitted

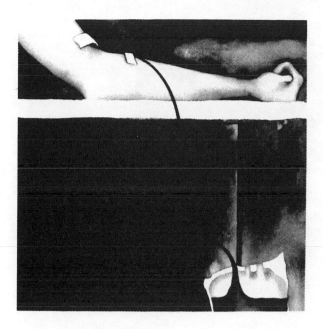

non-sexually from an infected person through a health or service provider to another person. Ordinary methods of disinfection for urine, stool and vomitus which are used for non-infected people are adequate for people who have AIDS or are carrying the AIDS virus. You may have wondered why your dentist wears gloves and perhaps a mask when treating you. This does not mean that he has AIDS or that he thinks you do. He is protecting you and himself from hepatitis, common colds or flu.

There is no danger in visiting a patient with AIDS or caring for him or her. Normal hygienic practices, like wiping of body fluid spills with a solution of water and household bleach (1 part household bleach to 10 parts water), will provide full protection.

Children in School None of the identified cases of AIDS in the United States are known or are suspected to have been transmitted from one child to another in school, day care, or foster care settings. Transmission would necessitate exposure of open cuts to the blood or other body fluids of the infected child, a highly unlikely occurrence. Even then routine safety procedures for handling blood or other body fluids

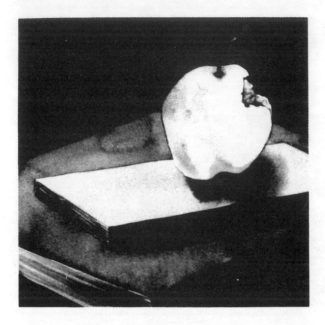

(which should be standard for all children in the school or day care setting) would be effective in preventing transmission from children with AIDS to other children in school.

Children with AIDS are highly susceptible to infections, such as chicken pox, from other children. Each child with AIDS should be examined by a doctor before attending school or before returning to school, day care or foster care settings after an illness. No blanket rules can be made for all school boards to cover all possible cases of children with AIDS and each case should be considered separately and individualized to the child and the setting, as would be done with any child with a special problem, such as cerebral palsy or asthma. A good team to make such decisions with the schoolboard would be the child's parents, physician and a public health official.

Casual social contact between children and persons infected with the AIDS virus is not dangerous.

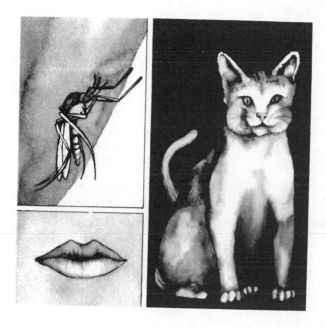

Insects   There are no known cases of AIDS transmission by insects, such as mosquitoes.

Pets   Dogs, cats and domestic animals are not a source of infection from AIDS virus.

Tears and Saliva   Although the AIDS virus has been found in tears and saliva, no instance of transmission from these body fluids has been reported.

AIDS comes from sexual contacts with infected persons and from the sharing of syringes and needles. There is no danger of infection with AIDS virus by casual social contact.

Testing of Military Personnel   You may wonder why the Department of Defense is currently testing its uniformed services personnel for presence of the AIDS virus antibody. The military feel this procedure is necessary because the uniformed services act as their own blood bank in a time of national emergency. They also need to protect new recruits (who unknowingly may be AIDS virus carriers) from receiving live virus vaccines. These vaccines could activate disease and be potentially life-threatening to the recruits.

AIDS: what is currently understood

Although AIDS is still a mysterious disease in many ways, our scientists have learned a great deal about it. In five years we know more about AIDS than many diseases that we have studied for even longer periods. While there is no vaccine or cure, the results from the health and behavioral research community can only add to our knowledge and increase our understanding of the disease and ways to prevent and treat it.

In spite of all that is known about transmission of the AIDS virus, scientists will learn more. One possibility is the potential discovery of factors that may better explain the mechanism of AIDS infection.

Why are the antibodies produced by the body to fight the AIDS virus not able to destroy that virus?

The antibodies detected in the blood of carriers of the AIDS virus are ineffective, at least when classic AIDS is actually triggered. They cannot check the damage caused by the virus, which is by then present in large numbers in the body. Researchers cannot explain this important observation. We still do not know why the AIDS virus is not destroyed by man's immune system.

Summary

AIDS no longer is the concern of any one segment of society; it is the concern of us all. No American's life is in danger if he/she or their sexual partners do not engage in high risk sexual behavior or use shared needles or syringes to inject illicit drugs into the body.

People who engage in high risk sexual behavior or who shoot drugs are risking infection with the AIDS virus and are risking their lives and the lives of others, including their unborn children.

We cannot yet know the full impact of AIDS on our society. From a clinical point of view, there may be new manifestations of AIDS—for

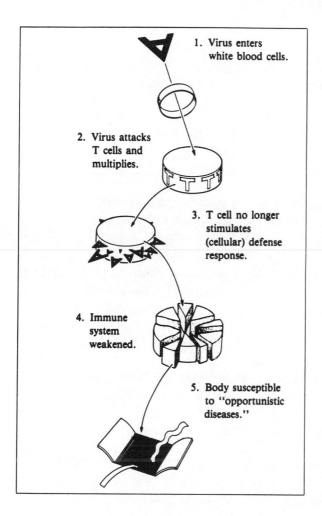

1. Virus enters white blood cells.

2. Virus attacks T cells and multiplies.

3. T cell no longer stimulates (cellular) defense response.

4. Immune system weakened.

5. Body susceptible to "opportunistic diseases."

example, mental disturbances due to the infection of the brain by the AIDS virus in carriers of the virus. From a social point of view, it may bring to an end the free-wheeling sexual lifestyle which has been called the sexual revolution. Economically, the care of AIDS patients will put a tremendous strain on our already overburdened and costly health care delivery system.

The most certain way to avoid getting the AIDS virus and to control the AIDS epidemic in the United States is for individuals to avoid promiscuous sexual practices, to maintain mutually faithful monogamous sexual relationships and to avoid injecting illicit drugs.

Look to the Future

The Challenge of the Future   An enormous challenge to public health lies ahead of us and we would do well to take a look at the future. We must be prepared to manage those things we can predict, as well as those we cannot.

At the present time there is no vaccine to prevent AIDS. There is no cure. AIDS, which can be transmitted sexually and by sharing needles and syringes among illicit intravenous drug users, is bound to produce profound changes in our society, changes that will affect us all.

Information and Education Only Weapons Against AIDS   It is estimated that in 1991 54,000 people will die from AIDS. At this moment, many of them are not infected with the AIDS virus. With proper information and education, as many as 12,000 to 14,000 people could be saved in 1991 from death by AIDS.

AIDS will Impact All   The changes in our society will be economic and political and will affect our social institutions, our educational practices, and our health care. Although AIDS may never touch you personally, the societal impact certainly will.

Be Educated—Be Prepared   Be prepared. Learn as much about AIDS as you can. Learn to separate scientific information from rumor and myth. The Public Health Service, your local public health officials and your family physician will be able to help you.

Concern About Spread of AIDS   While the concentration of AIDS cases is in the larger urban areas today, it has been found in every state and with the mobility of our society, it is likely that cases of AIDS will appear far and wide.

Special Education Concerns   There are a number of people, primarily adolescents, that do not yet know they will be homosexual or become drug abusers and will not heed this message; there are others who are illiterate and cannot heed this message. They must be reached and taught the risk behaviors that expose them to infection with the AIDS virus.

High Risk Get Blood Test   The greatest public health problem lies in the large number of individuals with a history of high risk behavior who have been infected with and may be spreading the AIDS virus. Those with high risk behavior must be encouraged to protect others by adopting safe sexual practices and by the use of clean equipment for intravenous drug use. If a blood test for antibodies to the AIDS virus is necessary to get these individuals to use safe sexual practices, they should get a blood test. Call your local health department for information on where to get the test.

Anger and Guilt   Some people afflicted with AIDS will feel a sense of anger and others a sense of guilt. In spite of these understandable reactions, everyone must join the effort to control the epidemic, to provide for the care of those with AIDS, and to do all we can to inform and educate others about AIDS, and how to prevent it.

Confidentiality   Because of the stigma that has been associated with AIDS, many afflicted with the disease or who are infected with the AIDS virus are reluctant to be identified with AIDS. Because there is no vaccine to prevent AIDS and no cure, many feel there is nothing to be gained by revealing sexual contacts that might also be infected with the AIDS virus. When a community or a state requires reporting of those infected with the AIDS virus to public health authorities in order to trace sexual and intravenous drug contacts—as is the practice with other sexually transmitted diseases—those infected with the AIDS virus go underground out of the mainstream of health care and education. For this reason current public health practice is to protect the privacy of the individual infected with the AIDS virus and to maintain the strictest confidentiality concerning his/her health records.

State and Local AIDS Task Forces   Many state and local jurisdictions where AIDS has been seen in the greatest numbers have AIDS task forces with heavy representation from the field of public health joined by others who can speak broadly to issues of access to care, provision of care and the availability of community and psychiatric support services. Such a task force is needed in every community with the power to develop plans and policies, to speak, and to act for the good of the public health at every level.

State and local task forces should plan ahead and work collaboratively with other jurisdictions to reduce transmission of AIDS by far-reaching informational and educational programs. As AIDS impacts more strongly on society, they should be charged with making recommendations to provide for the needs of those afflicted with AIDS. They also will be in the best position to answer the concerns and direct the activities of those who are not infected with the AIDS virus.

The responsibility of State and local task forces should be far reaching and might include the following areas:

- Insure enforcement of public health regulation of such practices as ear piercing and tattooing to prevent transmission of the AIDS virus.

- Conduct AIDS education programs for police, firemen, correctional institution workers and emergency medical personnel for dealing with AIDS victims and the public.

- Insure that institutions catering to children or adults who soil themselves or their surroundings with urine, stool, and vomitus have adequate equipment for cleanup and disposal, and have policies to insure the practice of good hygiene.

School   Schools will have special problems in the future. In addition to the guidelines already mentioned in this pamphlet, there are other things that should be considered such as sex education and education of the handicapped.

Sex Education   Education concerning AIDS must start at the lowest grade possible as part of any health and hygiene program. The appearance of AIDS could bring together diverse groups of parents and educators with opposing views on inclusion of sex education in the curricula. There is now no doubt that we need sex education in schools and that it must include information on heterosexual and homosexual relationships. The threat of AIDS should be sufficient to permit a sex education curriculum with a heavy emphasis on prevention of AIDS and other sexually transmitted diseases.

Handicapped and Special Education   Children with AIDS or ARC will be attending school along with others who carry the AIDS virus. Some children will develop brain disease which will produce changes in mental behavior. Because of the right to special education of the handicapped and the mentally retarded, school boards and higher authorities will have to provide guidelines for the management of such children on a case-by-case basis.

Labor and Management   Labor and management can do much to prepare for AIDS so that misinformation is kept to a minimum. Unions should issue preventive health messages because many employees will listen more carefully to a union message than they will to one from public health authorities.

AIDS Education at the Work Site   Offices, factories, and other work sites should have a plan in operation for education of the work force and accommodation of AIDS or ARC patients *before* the first such case appears at the work site. Employees with AIDS or ARC should be dealt with as are any workers with a chronic illness. In-house video programs provide an excellent source of education and can be individualized to the needs of a specific work group.

Strain on the Health Care Delivery System   The health care system in many places will be overburdened as it is now in urban areas with large numbers of AIDS patients. It is predicted that during 1991 there will be 145,000 patients requiring hospitalization at least once and 54,000 patients who will die of AIDS. Mental disease (dementia) will occur in some patients who have the AIDS virus before they have any other manifestation such as ARC or classic AIDS.

State and local task forces will have to plan for these patients by utilizing conventional and time honored systems but will also have to investigate alternate methods of treatment and alternate sites for care including home-care.

The strain on the health system can be lessened by family, social, and psychological support mechanisms in the community. Programs are needed to train chaplains, clergy, social workers, and volunteers to deal with AIDS. Such support is particularly critical to the minority communities.

Mental Health   Our society will also face an additional burden as we better understand the mental health implications of infection by the AIDS virus. Upon being informed of infection with the AIDS virus, a young, active, vigorous person faces anxiety and depression brought on by fears associated with social isolation, illness, and dying. Dealing with these individual and family concerns will require the best efforts of mental health professionals.

Controversial Issues   A number of controversial AIDS issues have arisen and will continue to be debated largely because of lack of knowledge about AIDS, how it is spread, and how it can be prevented. Among these are the issues of compulsory blood testing, quarantine, and identification of AIDS carriers by some visible sign.

Compulsory Blood Testing   Compulsory blood testing of individuals is not necessary. The procedure could be unmanageable and cost prohibitive. It can be expected that many who *test* negatively might actually be positive due to *recent* exposure to the AIDS virus and give a false sense of security to the individual and his/her sexual partners concerning necessary protective behavior. The prevention behavior described in this report, if adopted, will protect the American public and contain the AIDS epidemic. Voluntary testing will be available to those who have been involved in high risk behavior.

Quarantine   Quarantine has no role in the management of AIDS because AIDS is not spread by casual contact. The only time that some form of quarantine might be indicated is in a situation where an individual carrying the AIDS virus knowingly and willingly continues to expose others through sexual contact or sharing drug equipment. Such circumstances should be managed on a case-by-case basis by local authorities.

Identification of AIDS Carriers by Some Visible Sign   Those who suggest the marking of carriers of the AIDS virus by some visible sign have not thought the matter through thoroughly. It would require testing of the entire population which is unnecessary, unmanageable and costly. It would miss those recently infected individuals who would test negatively, but be infected. The entire procedure would give a false sense of security. AIDS must and will be treated as a disease that can infect anyone. AIDS should not be used as an excuse to discriminate against any group or individual.

Updating Information   As the Surgeon General, I will continually monitor the most current and accurate health, medical, and scientific information and make it available to you, the American people. Armed with this information you can join in the discussion and resolution of AIDS-related issues that are critical to your health, your children's health, and the health of the nation.

Additional Information
Telephone Hotlines
(Toll Free)
PHS AIDS Hotline
800-342-AIDS
800-342-2437

National Sexually Transmitted Diseases Hotline/American Social Health
  Association
800-227-8922

National Gay Task Force
AIDS Information Hotline
800-221-7044
(212) 807-6016 (NY State)

Information Sources
U.S. Public Health Service
Public Affairs Office
Hubert H. Humphrey Building, Room 725-H
200 Independence Avenue, S.W.
Washington, D.C. 20201
Phone: (202) 245-6867

Local Red Cross or American Red Cross
AIDS Education Office
1730 D Street, N.W.
Washington, D.C. 20006
Phone: (202) 737-8300

American Association of Physicians for Human Rights
P.O. Box 14366
San Francisco, CA 94114
Phone: (415) 558-9353

AIDS Action Council
729 Eighth Street, S.E., Suite 200
Washington, D.C. 20003
Phone: (202) 547-3101

Gay Men's Health Crisis
P.O. Box 274
132 West 24th Street
New York, NY 10011
Phone: (212) 807-6655

Hispanic AIDS Forum
c/o APRED
853 Broadway, Suite 2007
New York, NY 10003
Phone: (212) 870-1902 or 870-1864

Los Angeles AIDS Project
1362 Santa Monica Boulevard
Los Angeles, California 90046
(213) 871-AIDS

Minority Task Force on AIDS
c/o New York City Council of Churches
475 Riverside Drive, Room 456
New York, NY 10115
Phone: (212) 749-1214

Mothers of AIDS Patients (MAP)
c/o Barbara Peabody
3403 E Street
San Diego, CA 92102
(619) 234-3432

National AIDS Network
729 Eighth Street, S.E., Suite 300
Washington, D.C. 20003
(202) 546-2424

National Association of People with AIDS
P.O. Box 65472
Washington, D.C. 20035
(202) 483-7979

National Coalition of Gay Sexually Transmitted Disease Services
c/o Mark Behar
P.O. Box 239
Milwaukee, WI 53201
Phone: (414) 277-7671

National Council of Churches/AIDS Task Force
475 Riverside Drive, Room 572
New York, NY 10115
Phone: (212) 870-2421

San Francisco AIDS Foundation
333 Valencia Street, 4th Floor
San Francisco, CA 94103
Phone: (415) 863-2437

RESOURCES

U. S. AIDS Information Hotline Numbers.

National AIDS Hotline	(800) 342-AIDS
Alabama	(800) 455-3741
Alaska	(800) 478-2437
Arizona	(800) 334-1540
Arkansas	(800) 445-7720
California	
Northern California	(800) FOR-AIDS
Southern California	(800) 922-AIDS
Colorado	(303) 331-8305
Connecticut	(203) 566-1157
Delaware	(302) 995-8422
District of Columbia	(202) 332-AIDS
Florida	(800) FLA-AIDS
Georgia	(800) 551-2728
Hawaii	(808) 922-1313
Idaho	(208) 334-5944
Illinois	(800) AID-AIDS
Indiana	(317) 633-8406
Iowa	(800) 532-3301
Kansas	(800) 232-0040
Kentucky	(800) 654-AIDS
Louisiana	(800) 992-4379
Maine	(800) 851-AIDS
Maryland	(800) 638-6252
Massachusetts	(800) 235-2331
Minnesota	(800) 248-AIDS
Mississippi	(800) 826-2961
Montana	(406) 252-1212
Nebraska	(800) 782-2437

Nevada
  Reno . . . . (702) 329–AIDS
  Las Vegas . . . . (702) 383–1393
New Jersey . . . . (800) 624–2377
New Mexico . . . . (505) 827–0006
New York . . . . (800) 462–1884
North Carolina . . . . (919) 733–7301
North Dakota . . . . (800) 592–1861
Ohio . . . . (800) 332–AIDS
Oklahoma . . . . (405) 271–6434
Oregon . . . . (503) 229–5792
Pennsylvania . . . . (800) 692–7254
Rhode Island . . . . (402) 227–6502
South Carolina . . . . (800) 332–AIDS
South Dakota . . . . (800) 472–2180
Tennessee . . . . (800) 342–AIDS
Texas
  Dallas . . . . (214) 559–AIDS
  Houston . . . . (713) 524–AIDS
Utah . . . . (800) 843–9388
Vermont . . . . (800) 882–AIDS
West Virginia . . . . (800) 642–8244
Wisconsin . . . . (800) 334–AIDS
Wyoming . . . . (307) 777–7953

Major Organizational Resources

American Foundation for AIDS
  Research
40 W. 57th Street, Suite 406
New York, NY 10019

American Medical Association
535 North Dearborn Street
Chicago, IL 60610

American Red Cross
430 17th Street, N.W.
Washington, D.C. 20006

National Leadership Coalition on
  AIDS
1150 17th Street, N.W.
Washington, D.C. 20036

The Surgeon General's Report
U. S. Public Health Service
P. O. Box 23961
Washington, D.C. 20026

The San Francisco AIDS
  Foundation
25 Van Ness Avenue
San Francisco CA 94102
Telephone (415) 864-4376

Service Employees International
  Union
A.F.L. - C.I.O.
1313 L Street, N.W.
Washington, D.C. 20005
Telephone (202) 898-2300

Minority Task Force on AIDS
New York City Council of
  Churches
475 Riverside Drive
New York, NY 10015
Telephone (212) 749-1214

National AIDS Network
729 Eighth Street, S.E.
Washington, D.C. 20003
Telephone (202) 564-2424

Gay Men's Health Crisis
354 W. 18th Street
New York, NY 10011
Telephone (212) 547-3101

AIDS Project Los Angeles
7362 Santa Monica Boulevard
Los Angeles CA 90046
Telephone (213) 876-AIDS

AIDS Action Committee
661 Boylston Street
Boston, MA 02116
Telephone (617) 437-6200

Minnesota AIDS Project
2025 Nicollett Avenue
  South #200
Minneapolis, MN 55404
Telephone (612) 870-7773

National Gay Task Force
AIDS Information Hotline
Telephone (800) 221-7044

Resources Outside the United States

CANADA

AIDS Vancouver
1033 Davie Street
Vancouver, B.C.

Centretown Community Resources
100 Argyle Avenue
Ottawa, Ontario

AIDS Committee of Toronto
556 Church Street
Toronto, Ontario

Comite SIDA du Quebec
3757 rue Prud'homme
Montreal, Quebec

MEXICO

CONA SIDA
Ministry of Health
Mexico, D.F.

PUERTO RICO

Fundacion AIDS de P.R.
Call Box AIDS
Louisa Street Station
San Juan, P.R. 00914

AUSTRALIA/NEW ZEALAND

National AIDS Coordinating
    Committee
Commonwealth Department of
    Health
P. O. Box 100
Woden 06, Australia

New Zealand AIDS Foundation
Auckland Hospital
Auckland, New Zealand

Victorian AIDS Council
P. O. Box 174 Richmond
Melbourne 3121, Australia

EUROPE

Terrence Higgins Trust
BM AIDS
London, WCIN, England

Deutsch AIDS-Hilfe
Neibuhrstrasse 71
1000 Berlin 12, W. Germany

AIDS Policy Coordination
Burgo GVO
Prins Hendricklaan 12
1075 BB Amsterdam, Holland

SIDA STUDI
Bruc, 26, prol
08010 Barcelona, Spain

Index